Praise for CAL OREY's
Classic Health Books

The Healing Powers of Superfoods
"Ancient healing wisdom meets modern-day foods in this super book."
—Ann Louise Gittleman, Ph.D., C.N.S.,
author of *The Fat Flush Plan*

"In *The Healing Powers of Superfoods*, we're thankfully
rediscovering these amazingly healthy foods again today."
—Will Clower, Ph.D., CEO, Mediterranean Wellness

The Healing Powers of Tea
"Confirmed enthusiasts of the drink will most appreciate Orey's
well-constructed and comprehensive guide; foodies and those
with an interest in alternative-health therapies will also want
to thumb through it."
—*Publishers Weekly*

"Tea is an ancient elixir that is making quite a therapeutic
comeback. I know this book will be your cup of tea!"
—Ann Louise Gittleman, Ph.D., C.N.S.,
author of *The Fat Flush Plan*

"*The Healing Powers of Tea*, like the drink itself, is a
nourishing comfort."
—Will Clower, Ph.D., CEO, Mediterranean Wellness

The Healing Powers of Vinegar, *Revised and Updated*
"A practical, health-oriented book that everyone who wants to stay
healthy and live longer should read."
—Patricia Bragg, N.D., Ph.D., author of *Apple Cider Vinegar*

"For heart, mind, and body, Cal Orey shows us why coffee is the most comforting health food on the planet."
—Dr. Will Clower, Ph.D., CEO, Mediterranean Wellness

The Healing Powers of Honey
"A fascinating read about a natural remedy that is a rich source of antioxidants."
—Ray Sahelian, M.D., author of *Mind Boosters*

"Not everyone can be a beekeeper, but Cal Orey shares the secrets that honeybees and their keepers have always known. Honey is good for body and soul."
—Kim Flottum, editor of *Bee Culture* magazine and author of several honeybee books

The Healing Powers of Chocolate
"The right kind, the right amount of chocolate may just save your life."
—Ann Louise Gittleman, Ph.D., C.N.S., author of *The Fat Flush Plan*

"Chocolate is a taste of divine ecstasy on Earth. It is our sensual communion. Orey's journalistic style and efforts share this insight with readers around the world."
—Jim Walsh, founder, Intentional Chocolate

Books by Cal Orey

The Healing Powers of Herbs and Spices

The Healing Powers of Essential Oils

The Healing Powers of Superfoods

The Healing Powers of Tea

The Healing Powers of Coffee

The Healing Powers of Honey

The Healing Powers of Chocolate

The Healing Powers of Olive Oil

The Healing Powers of Vinegar

202 Pets' Peeves

Doctors' Orders

Available from Kensington Publishing Corp.

The
Healing Powers of
Herbs and Spices

A COMPLETE GUIDE TO NATURE'S MOST MAGICAL MEDICINE

Cal Orey

CITADEL PRESS
Kensington Publishing Corp.
www.kensingtonbooks.com

CITADEL PRESS BOOKS are published by

Kensington Publishing Corp.
119 West 40th Street
New York, NY 10018

All Kensington titles, imprints, and distributed lines are available at special quantity discounts for bulk purchases for sales promotions, premiums, fund-raising, educational, or institutional use. Special book excerpts or customized printings can also be created to fit specific needs. For details, write or phone the office of the Kensington sales manager: Kensington Publishing Corp., 119 West 40th Street, New York, NY 10018, attn: Sales Department; phone 1-800-221-2647.

CITADEL PRESS and the Citadel logo are Reg. U.S. Pat. & TM Off.

ISBN-13: 978-0-8065-4048-1
ISBN-10: 0-8065-4048-6

First trade paperback printing: January 2021

10 9 8 7 6 5 4 3 2 1

Printed in the United States of America

Electronic edition:

ISBN-13: 978-0-8065-4049-8 (e-book)
ISBN-10: 0-8065-4049-4 (e-book)

A *special dedication*...

This book is dedicated to Mediterranean herbs and spices. Ancient and aromatic bay (laurel) leafed trees and garlic fields are my muse in California. Whenever a wanderlust spirit lures me away from the Golden State, seasonings in different regions connect me to family and home.

CONTENTS

Foreword

SEASONINGS ABOARD

This is not a memory or a dream. I documented my real-life sea journeys before setting sail. New countries, new cuisines, and exciting herbs and spices were part of the plan. This is one of my journal entries. It is penned in past tense: words from the heart. These are my true feelings about our daring voyage—me, my beloved wife, and chief mate, Dottie—before we embarked on one of many sailing adventures . . .

I made the food on my 46-foot boat, the sailing vessel *Amari*. I was very particular about having cinnamon at the ready for an ocean passage squash soup, tarragon for a quick tuna salad lunch, and fennel for that impromptu marinara for pasta. These seasonings are absolute necessities aboard, whether we were in water in the eastern Caribbean islands or en route to Spain. We were prepping her, a ship to go 3,600 miles across the Atlantic Ocean and into the Mediterranean for five months.

Just ashore in Brewers Bay was a local food vendor who had set up shop just down from the University of the Virgin Islands. Walking downwind of his place, I caught a scent that had me sniffing like a puppy, eager to investigate immediately.

This man had a bright face, a ready smile, and was selling Spicy Jamaican Patties, which are very traditional to these islands. They're basically a fold-over of dough with filling. I know. It sounds a bit boring. But oh my, after biting into one the flavors exploded in my mouth.

A CARNIVAL OF DELICIOUS SPICES

Because I'm a science geek, I made it my mission to reverse engineer the patties so I could make something similar back on the boat. But I couldn't dissect it. What I got from this simple patty was a carnival of delectable spices, a love-in of perhaps allspice, cinnamon, ginger, nutmeg, and/or cloves. Not to forget fresh garlic and thyme. I tried to figure out what was in there, but it was just too much. I gave up and looked up at him like he was Gandalf or Dumbledore and pleaded with him to tell me, "How did you do this?"

He laughed and then told me what I was eating wasn't his, but his mastery of spice balance came to him from his mother and hers before him. The spices that define his culture of food and flavor stretch back, he said, to the first days of the Carib. Unwritten recipes of understanding that came to define the flavors of these islands. They became the flavors of their food, family, and lives, woven into the threads of their cultural tapestry.

We will arrive in the Mediterranean to sample the food cultures that spill out of this region, so famous for its food and also its health. Just as in the Caribbean, the rich culture of spices, herbs, and flavors not only defines the residents' food, but also who they are.

CRUISING TO THE MEDITERRANEAN FLAVORS

After moving through the Azores and landing in Lagos, Portugal, it would be time to explore the flavors of this amazing region. By the time we'd make landfall, I expected to be so grateful to reach port. We'll be keying into the herbs and spices that make the local food magical: the sweet paprika, cinnamon, and bay leaf.

After the survey of Portugal, we will move just inside the Straits of Gibraltar, along the amazing coast of Spain, where cooks lace saffron and paprika into their delicate savory paella — and other dishes! My wife Dottie and I have a friend in Valencia who actually has a paella hut dedicated to this one dish!

Our ground plan is to visit the French Côte d'Azur and sample their traditional use of garlic, tarragon, and fennel, which are legendary. Before returning home in fall, the strategy is to cruise our way down the Italian coastline, sampling their pungent basil, oregano, and thyme.

In some ways traveling felt like the seafaring groups of ages past, who found life-altering spices on the shores of new locations. These discoveries led to the creation of trade routes that opened up not only these amazing flavors, but entire cultures to the world. It's a gift, in my mind, to be able to sample the herbs and spices that played such an important role in the past.

THE HEALTHIEST CULTURES ON THE PLANET

Many cultures use herbs and spices because they're delicious, but these cooking essentials may contribute to the fact that the eating habits of the Mediterranean are among the healthiest on the planet. Their health advantage is what intrigued me to write books based on the Mediterranean approach to diet.

As a bonus, the same spices that Mediterranean cooks add to soups, sauces, and salads made their food as delicious as it is healthy. Using these herbs and spices to flavor your food will alleviate the cravings for the extra salt, sugar, and processed food products that contribute to the chronic disease symptoms.

Other cultures learned about herbs and spices through centuries of experience, building their cultural knowledge over generations. But now through Cal Orey's most recent work, *The Healing Powers of Herbs and Spices*, you can understand these same simple-yet-potent plants in a way that gives you access to them in your home and daily life.

This book provides direct access to this understanding, so you can get to know the spices, learn the herbs, and understand how to apply them to your health and hearth every day.

—Will Clower, Ph.D.
CEO, Mediterranean Wellness

Introduction

Welcome to my world of herbs and spices.

As a seasoned (pun intended) nutrition journalist-author I've cultivated an aromatic garden of savvy sources to provide a fresh perspective. As a health enthusiast with a knack to simplify technical jargon, I have embraced the topic of herbs and spices.

For two decades, as the creator of the *Healing Powers* series, I've dished on herbs and spices. Yes, my books about vinegar, olive oil, honey, chocolate, coffee, tea, and superfoods all included wisdom about herbs and spices. But I have not isolated and provided comprehensive information on these dozens of different and remarkable nature's seasonings—until now! With these seasonings serving as my tour guides through foreign territory, I tackled the plant-based world of scientific studies, health advantages, folk remedies, beauty secrets, and culinary recipes. The subject of ancient herbs and spices is a hot topic in the twenty-first century. Like a passionate poet at the helm of the vessel, I will be your captain on a cruise to explore a worldly topic—herbs and spices!

I'm taking you on a gastronomic, super sensory, and healing adventure. Close your eyes and think of a faraway land; chances are the herb or spice you read about in this book has roots there. Imagine old-time explorers like Christopher Columbus who were brave enough to cross oceans to find and bring back nature's greatest treasures—herbs and spices. You, too, may feel the urge to find and savor a new adventure in flavor.

So, come along. Take the plunge into *The Healing Powers of Herbs and Spices*. It is authentic. And I infuse a whole lot of enthusiasm and season it up for zest. Anchors aweigh!

Author's Note

It's here—the ninth book in the *Healing Powers* series, a new book with a serious wow factor. I believe each chapter will inspire you to add to your collection of herbs and spices. This book is meant to be enjoyed and used as a reference tool. It does not provide medical advice.

Be sure to consult your doctor or healthcare specialist before using any herb or spice that you haven't tried before. True, nature's herbs and spices are natural, but that doesn't mean they are not potent when consumed or used topically. It is advised to do a skin patch test if used topically; and definitely, for safety's sake, use less rather than more when you try them. Food allergies can occur even with herbs and spices. Be sure to heed the Safety Sound Bites you'll find here!

The recipes in this book are varied. Many are dishes are from the twentieth century, but I've given them a twenty-first-century healthful twist. The dishes are tested by me, my family and friends, and/or chefs, herbs and spices companies, and big-name superfood houses and organizations. You can adjust the number of herbs and spices in the recipes to fit your tastes and needs.

You will be surprised by the colors, flavors, textures, and healing powers of plants. Brew a cup of herbal tea, go to chapter 1 or skip ahead to a chapter that tempts you. This book can be read like a novel or used as a reference guide that allows you to flip to a specific topic. Either way, I trust you will revisit the pages, time after time.

PART 1

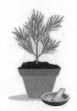

HERBS AND SPICES

The Spice of Life!

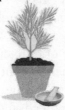

Variety's the very spice of life,
That gives it all its flavour.
—WILLIAM COWPER, "The Task"

I grew up in California surrounded by beautiful nature. The mountains and ocean were less than an hour's drive from our family home—which was a landscape garden suburbia. When my mom cooked and baked in the kitchen, the fragrant seasonings took my vivid imagination to faraway lands like Italy and France, places I saw on postcards she sent to me when she traveled abroad. And that is what ignited my love for European spices and herbs.

A TIME FOR HERBS AND SPICES

Centuries ago, Christopher Columbus chased the dream of discovering valuable seasonings like a hidden prize. Bold men sailed the seas to find a variety of herbs and spices, then bring them back home to share their riches.

Today, you can buy your herbs and spices at your local grocery store, online, at health food stores, and at farmers' markets. The chosen seasoning can be hidden in dishes you make or order when dining out. But priceless herbs and spices are still precious commodities, worthy of a lifetime of exploration. In this book you will set sail with me on an adventure into healthy living and flavorful dining as we discover, one by one, these amazing garden gifts.

Shortly after I began my book research, I found a big cardboard box on my doorstop—a gift from a friend. When I opened the package I was greeted by a strong wave of different aromas. The box was filled with dozens of individual packets containing a variety of herbs and spices. It was as if they were all saying, "Look at me! Choose me!" I took out each cellophane-wrapped and labeled packet. There were rows of small packages on my dining room table. Each one was filled with powders, pods, seeds, and stems—some familiar, some not.

I brought out a kit of glass bottles with stick-on labels that I had ordered online and went to work filling each container with a dried herb or spice. Foolishly, I did not wear a mask. My eyes began to water, and sniffles started. I sneezed several times. I was experiencing the potent compounds in the botanical plants. But I persevered!

Within a few hours, all my herbs and spices were inside the glass bottles and labeled. I was ready to arrange them in racks: a wrought iron spice rack to hang on the wall; an attractive stainless steel lazy Susan–type device for the kitchen corner; and two round wooden devices for inside the cool and dark kitchen cabinet. It was time to start my personal journey into the world of herbs and spices.

Two Terms, Two Definitions for Seasonings

Are herbs and spices different from each other? People—perhaps, you, too—often confuse the two words, since they have many of the same characteristics. And indeed, they are connected so it's no surprise, folks, even professional chefs use the two words interchangeably. After all, herbs and spices are both derived from aromatic plants. But, leafy herbs, like garlic and marjoram, come from the plant or leaves itself, while spices, such as allspice and nutmeg, come from the bark, flowers, roots, and seeds. To help you differentiate herbs and spices, remember that herbs come from fresh and dried leaves; spices from bark, flowers, fruit, seeds, and roots.

A PACKET OF HEALING POWERS

The chemical compounds in herbs and spices make them powerful gifts for your mind and body. They nourish our senses and provide wonderful memories, too. Think of the aroma and taste of eggnog with nutmeg during the holidays. Or the pungent flavor of garlic on pizza for a relaxing weekend night. But herbs and spices do much more.

Top doctors, nutritionists, chefs, and experts in the herbs and spices industry will tell you that the medical magic of herbs and spices is real.

"Herbs and spices are not just tasty flavor enhancers," author of *Radical Metabolism* health author Ann Louise Gittleman says. "They are loaded with healing phytonutrients straight from Mother Nature."

Health guru Jonny Bowden, Ph.D., author of the brilliant *150 Healthiest Foods on Earth, Revised Edition*, dishes more on "medicinal" herbs and spices. Like me, he gives credit to these workhorse wonders full of chemical compounds that can help lower the risks of facing heart disease, diabetes, obesity, and cancers.[1]

The Golden Door Cooks Light & Easy sophisticated author Chef Michel Stroot, whom I've interviewed in the past, notes in one of my favorite dog-eared timeless recipe books that fresh herbs are "an indispensable addition to the spa kitchen—and any other kitchen."[2]

Food experts, like these, know that herbs and spices provide a valuable chest of health benefits to mankind. The herbs in your fridge and the dried spices in your kitchen cupboard provide medicinal powers, home cures, weight loss benefits, beauty treatments, and adventurous flavors and textures to enhance plant-based dishes—the new "in" diet that will endure as long as people are interested in healthy eating.

PHYTONUTRIENTS ARE THE KEY

For more than five thousand years, nutrient-rich herbs and spices have been praised for their medicinal value, preserving and flavoring food and cosmetics, and preventing and curing illnesses. Simply put, phytonutrients—the medical term for the chemical components in botanical products—have been providing a multitude of healing virtues and vibes for a long, long time.

While the health perks of herbs and spices go back to biblical times (some herbalists and historians say fifty thousand years!), we now better understand how they work and offer their healing powers. Today, scientists are finding how phytochemical-rich herbs and spices can help lower the risk of developing heart disease, cancer, and other health ailments that can boost our well-being and longevity.

ORAC VALUES OF HERBS AND SPICES

Herbalists and medical researchers refer to herbs and spices as superfoods. They are listed in the ORAC ranking, like nutrient-rich fruits and vegetables. ORAC is an acronym for the Oxygen Radical Absorbance Capacity, a guideline that shows how many antioxidants are in a seasoning. The higher the number, the higher the amount of good-for-you nutrients are in an herb or spice.

Take a look below at several herbs and spices, listed from A–Z, which have healing properties when eaten or used topically. The ranking number listed specifically shows you the amount of antioxidants in these super seasonings.

Cilantro-Fresh	1 tablespoon	510
Cloves	½ teaspoon	7,861
Cumin	½ teaspoon	1,920
Garlic	½ teaspoon	725
Marjoram	½ teaspoon	675
Oregano	½ teaspoon	5,000
Paprika	½ teaspoon	450
Parsley	½ teaspoon	1,850

Tarragon	1 teaspoon	777
Thyme	½ teaspoon	688
Turmeric	½ teaspoon	3,975

(Source: Data from U.S. Department of Agriculture)

Researchers writing in the *Journal of the Association of Official Analytical Chemists* discovered how herbs and spices were praised for their past and present culinary and medicinal purposes. Their article also acknowledged that herbs and spices can protect you from acute and chronic diseases. It revealed fascinating evidence that herbs and spices contain antioxidant, anti-inflammatory, anti-tumorigenic, anti-carcinogenic, and glucose-cholesterol benefits as well as properties that affect mind and mood. Most importantly, specific properties were applauded, including sulfur-containing compounds, tannins, alkaloids, phenolic diterpenes, and vitamins, especially flavonoids and polyphenols.[3]

Herbs and spices, including, clove, garlic, oregano, sage, and turmeric (some of my Mediterranean favorites), were found to contain excellent sources of antioxidants with their high content of phenolic compounds. Also, it was noted that use of spices was connected to a lower risk of death from heart and respiratory system diseases and cancer. But the actual role of herbs and spices in the preventive health care is still unclear. Which herb or spice was given sole credit for lowering the risk of developing cancer? Nobody knows for sure. All the more reason to stock up your spice rack and fridge with a colorful variety to ensure you're covered![4]

CIAO, SEASONINGS

The *Healing Powers* series has featured the popular, heart-healthy Mediterranean diet and lifestyle for twenty years. This time, I'm giving top priority to the diet's herbs and spices that are found in the Oldways Mediterranean Diet pyramid foods chart. These seasonings include anise, bay leaf, clove, cumin, fennel, garlic, marjoram, oregano, parsley, pepper, tarragon, thyme, and zaatar.[5]

Also, the Mediterranean diet was reported by the *U.S. News and World Report* as the number one best diet for a third year in a row in 2020. Some of my 22 chosen herbs and spices, to praise chapter by chapter, have European roots, but others made their way to the Mediterranean countries via trace and usage for cuisine. These days, French dishes often include garlic, nutmeg, and thyme. Italian food includes those picks but also oregano, parsley, and sage. Garlic and thyme are popular in both countries. All of my choices can be and are used in Mediterranean foods.

An acquaintance told me she was glad that I'd be focusing on herbs and spices. She assumed I would be only addressing herbs and spices with roots from India, such as cardamom and turmeric. Yes, these non-European gifts do make the cut in this tome because they are used in Mediterranean cuisine, thanks to past and present supply and demand in European countries.

I prefer to mix it up. My recipe collection has an aromatic Mediterranean–West Coast twist. I often go back in my mind to my home in the Golden State where I was raised. The selection of the Mediterranean herbs and spices with roots in Europe are used in French and Italian cuisine.

As you can see in the ORAC chart, why these "superherbs" and "superspices" known as "functional foods" are healthy. It's due to the compounds and nutrients, according to herb and spice study scientists, suggesting hidden phytonutrients are what's behind the preventive nature of plants. Like nutrient-rich foods, the more variety of herbs you add to your diet, the more likely you are to achieve healing results.

The traditional well-balanced Mediterranean diet was based on the food preparation traditions of Crete, Greece, and southern Italy—in particular the diet of the poor people of the southern Mediterranean, which included nature's finest basic foods such as fruits and vegetables, beans and nuts, whole grains, fish, olive oil, small amount of sweets and red wine, water, and herbs and spices.

This selection of foods is linked to good health and longevity. It's a no-frills plant-based, balanced diet that continues to be ranked as one of the top U.S. healthiest diets in the twenty-first century.

I grew up eating these Mediterranean diet foods. However, like so many others, I also loved to indulge in fast food drive-thru and easy to heat it up frozen food. But as a rebellious, nature-loving baby boomer, when the seventies hit, I, like millions of others, discovered the benefits of eating health food. Enter plant power—herbs and spices to flavor up a vegan diet—rice and vegetables. So I came full circle, and to this day it's the balanced and seasoned Mediterranean dishes paired with herbs that I eat and want to share with you.

FRESH OR DRIED—OR BOTH?

Believe it or not, there is a fine art to usage of herbs in cooking and baking. You may wonder, "Do I use fresh or dried?" It depends. Living in California, a mecca of superfoods, I can tell you fresh herbs aren't always available or if they are, they can be pricey. And if these gems are store-bought the expiration date is like a ticking clock.

Woodier herbs, like oregano and thyme are fine used dried or fresh. Thyme, however, does make a pretty garnish. Some herbalists claim chives are best when fresh but sometimes, fresh herbs go to waste and into the trash. Dried herbs, a good quality and not expired, are convenient and more forgiving with usage of time. I can personally attest that using dried chives on a baked potato can suffice. But if on hand, I combine it with fresh Italian parsley for an extra punch, and ground black pepper. Also, you can use both fresh and dried varieties—for flavor and texture.

When cooking with fresh herbs, it's advised adding them at the end of cooking or baking a dish. You will maintain the integrity of flavor and good-for-you antioxidants. Dried herbs are concentrated and stronger in flavor. The rule of thumb is three-to-one formula. For instance, one teaspoon of dried thyme would equal one tablespoon fresh thyme. In the end, I vote for using both.

Nutritional Healing

Sweet Potato Pie

The first time I tasted sweet potato pie, I was traveling solo in the Deep South. I stopped at a small café on the outskirts of Atlanta, Georgia. The pastry was sweet-smelling and creamy, but something was missing. Years later, in my cabin, I made a homemade sweet potato and yam tart. It was good but not tasty either. The recipe below is a sweet and spicy find. It is one that finally got the flavoring right—thanks to the use of herbs and spices. It was created by my longtime central California friend, the co-owner of Sciabica's Olive Oil.

1 single pie crust pastry [You can make your own or
    use a store-bought variety and place it in a tart
    dish like I do]
¼ cup pecans, ground
2 tablespoons sugar

FILLING

3 sweet potatoes or yams, cooked (3 cups)
4 eggs
½ to ¾ cup brown sugar, packed (or pure maple syrup)
1 teaspoon cinnamon
½ teaspoon allspice or ginger
½ teaspoon nutmeg
1 teaspoon cloves, ground
1 teaspoon pure maple extract
½ teaspoon salt
1 tablespoon grated orange peel
1 cup evaporated milk (low fat)
1 teaspoon vanilla
1 tablespoon Marsala olive oil
Pecans for garnish

Preheat oven to 400 degrees Fahrenheit (F). Add nuts and sugar to pie crust. Roll out to fit a 10-inch pie tin; cut excess crust; flute edges. Place cooked sweet potatoes in mixing bowl, mash, add remaining ingredients: eggs, sugar, spices, orange peel, milk, vanilla, and olive oil. Whisk until blended. Pour mixture into prepared pie tin (lined with pastry). Cut 8 leaves out of excess pastry with leaf-shaped cookie cutter. Place on top of the filling. Bake for 15 minutes, lower heat to 350 degrees F, bake for another 35 to 40 minutes or until cake tester comes out clean from center of pie. Cover with foil loosely if browning too quickly. Serve with sweetened whipped cream and sprinkle with ground pecans or garnish with pecan halves. Author's note: When I made the pie, I substituted the evaporated milk with a mix of mascarpone cheese and half-and-half. I garnished the pie with thyme sprigs and star anise to take my taste buds and imagination to Italy.

Serves 8.

(Courtesy: Gemma Sanita Sciabica, *Cooking with California Olive Oil: Popular Recipes*)

Let's go back centuries ago, into the land of herbs and spices. It's time to discover how the real stories and some legends of people from all cultures and walks of life used botanical plants to flavor their food and enhance health.

HEALING HIGHLIGHTS FROM NATURE'S GARDEN-FEST

Including herbs and spices in your food and topically means that you're bringing disease-fighting antioxidants into your life. Healing powers include:

✓ Lowering your odds of facing heart disease . . . and holding on to healthy blood pressure and cholesterol numbers.

✓ Safeguarding the immune system to dodge colds, flu—and even cancer (nobody is immune).

✓ Revving up a sluggish metabolism to shed unwanted pounds (at any age!).

✓ Blocking inflammation—the scourge of health ailments and diseases.

✓ Easing aches, triggering feel-good endorphins (natural painkillers) in the body so you can enjoy limitless energy.

✓ Boosting mood to help you chillax and feel energized and happy.

✓ Gaining mental clarity, losing brain fog so you can revel in mindful pursuits at work or play.

✓ Adding quantity and quality years to your life and possibly even becoming an active centenarian!

Roots of Plant Power

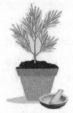

*But in truth, should I meet with gold or spices in great
quantity, I shall remain till I collect as much as
possible, and for this purpose I am proceeding solely in
quest of them.*
—CHRISTOPHER COLUMBUS

My first real-life adventure entering the world of herbs and spices goes
back to the summer. I was seven years old, living in San Jose,
California. We moved into a new house. My dad filled the yards with
trees, plants, flowers, and manicured lawns that looked like vibrant
green chives. One Saturday I had been swimming all day at a lodge
pool in the Los Gatos foothills. Lunch was grilled hamburgers with
spicy mustard and French fries sprinkled with salt and pepper—two
popular spices in the sixties. My best friend shared her anticipation of
an outdoor dinner awaiting at home. Sunburned, exhausted, and famished, I loved the idea of an evening meal to feed the senses but for me
it was a dream, not a reality.

"My mom worked today," I told my swimming pal, "so that means cold cuts from the take-out deli will be on our table."

When I walked into the house the stovetop was empty and kitchen table bare. Smelling sweet and savory aromas I followed the scent into the backyard. The grill was smoking hot, and barbecued pork chops with a cayenne and thyme rub were sizzling. On the wooden picnic table, I was greeted with toast spread with buttered minced garlic and parsley. Salad greens were drizzled with dill and fennel dressing from our small garden. I whiffed sweet potatoes with cinnamon sprinkled on top. The herbs and spices tasted like quintessential summertime picnic food. My mom and dad worked well together as a team for cookout dinners. It's the first time I remember distinctly smelling the symphony of spicy foods. The herbal fragrance lingered in the warm, sultry air.

That evening was more than a half a century ago, but the recollection lingers in my heart whenever I am around the herbs of my childhood. Now I enjoy travels to faraway lands where the spicy cuisine often connects me to home and family—and herbs and spices I savored on that magical Saturday.

Now, like a time traveler, I'm taking you with me centuries ago, to a time when aromatic herbs and spices were hidden riches, and finding them was like finding an oil well today.

HISTORICAL HEALING HERBS AND SPICES

During the stone age and biblical times, herbs and spices were put to work for their multipurpose benefits. Historians tell us that in the caveman days, people would use berries, roots, and seeds to season meat wrapped in plant leaves for cooking it. It was learned that this method provided and preserved flavor and health advantages, too. Artwork on pottery shows that spices were included in prehistoric cuisine. Archaeologists from Denmark, Germany, Spain, and the United Kingdom found proof of the use of spices at least seven thousand years ago. Europeans morphed from a hunters and gatherers lifestyle to one that included farming and growing herbs and spices.[1]

Other health researchers believe that archaeologists discovered evidence of herbs and spices as early as 50,000 B.C. Nobody knows for sure the exact date, but we do know seasonings have been around for a good long while!

Humans may have used the leaves of plants for flavoring meats around 2300 B.C., for wine making. In 330 B.C. spices were used by Asia, India, Greece, and Persian cultures...The spice trade flourished. Trade routes called the "Silk Road" (an ancient caravan route between China and the Mediterranean connecting the East and West) helped commerce to expand. Early records show herbs and spices were used for medicinal methods in ancient Egypt and Assyria and as food preservatives in ancient Rome and Greece. Documentation suggests herbs and spices were utilized during the Middle Ages for flavoring, food preservation, and medicinal purposes. Herbs and spices continued to spread in the 1800s as new trade routes expanded, making the commodities more affordable to use in a variety of European cultures.[2]

TIMELESS TREASURES, EIGHT ERAS

The region and time of events vary from historian to historian, herbalist to herbalist. Overall, the fact that herbs and spices made their way around the world is what matters. The history of each of my chosen herbs and spices provides pieces of the past. Take a glance at some data explaining how those herbs and spices you love to use evolved chronologically, century by century.

#1 Ancient Egypt: Since 3500 B.C., spices were multipurpose wonders used for flavoring food, in cosmetics, and in embalming the deceased. As the Egyptian empire expanded, spices attracted people in eastern Mediterranean countries. Spices helped preserve food, too. Spices were so valuable they were used as a form of payment throughout many regions and centuries. Herbs, like spices, were also praised for their healing powers.

#2 Age-Old Asia-Mesopotamia: Spices made their way into China, thanks to the Moluccas. It is believed that during the fifth century, ginger plants were found growing in pots and brought along on boats sailing in the seas between China and Southeast Asia. The herb and spices were used to aid in health and to stave off diseases like scurvy, which is caused by a vitamin C deficiency. Herbs and spices were used in different civilizations during ancient Mesopotamia, which is an area of Southwest Asia, rich in botanical plants.

#3 Early India: By the eighth century B.C., herbs and spices are believed to have been used for both enriching the flavor of food and helping achieve better health. Some of these spices, which were part of the Ayurvedic medicine (ancient Indian medicine for the body and mind), included cardamom, cumin, and turmeric—healing spices I discuss in this book.

#4 Historic Greece and Rome: In Greece, a variety of spices and herbs—particularly caraway, coriander, and fennel—were used in cooking. And let's not forget the popularity of the herbs garlic and parsley, believed to have medicinal advantages. Greeks used herbs as crowns for leaders and heroes. Romans believed herbs had magical powers.

#5 Ageless Arabia: During ancient times to A.D. 1096, trading of spices was from Arabia. The source of the spices was secret knowledge from other countries because it gave the Arabians more power. Other cultures, such as the Greeks and Romans, also didn't know the origin of spices. Later, doctors used them for their medicinal benefits.

#6 Middle Ages: During the Middle Ages, growing herbs and studying their medicinal benefits were popular pastimes for royalty, commoners, and clergymen. Asian spices were used by European royalty because they were so costly. Spices such as ginger, saffron, and pepper were incredibly expensive, just as gold is to us today. But once the Crusades period arrived (a time of wars from 1095 to the sixteenth century), international trade brought the prices down for spices, making their usage more widespread, not just for royalty. In time, medical practitioners provided the healing benefits of spices and herbs for people of all classes.

The Age of Spice Discovery

From the 1400s to 1600s, explorers set sail to discover riches—herbs and spices, priceless commodities. You, like me, probably played the hide-and-seek swimming pool game "Marco Polo." More than five hundred years ago, men like Christopher Columbus, Ferdinand Magellan, and Marco Polo traveled the seas in search of hidden herbs and spices. Instead of the kid's pool game Marco Polo to find a person, imagine the courage of the European explorers who sought their fortunes, hoping to find herbs and spices in faraway lands. The healing herbs and spices they discovered would be used to flavor food and preserve it, for medicinal purposes, and to help guard people against the deadly bubonic plague in the Middle Ages. Historians share that in the 1600s European nations started trading posts in Asia. This, in turn, made spices more available to Mediterranean countries.

#7 Early Colonial Europe and America: The United States started entering the spice trade in the 1700s. When spices grew more in demand their cost began to decline. From the 1800s on, herbs and spices were used in culinary dishes as well as for medicinal purposes. Common ailments, from digestion woes to respiratory issues, were dealt with by putting herbs and spices to work to help stave off discomfort. During the Colonial period in the nineteenth century, a busy pepper trade exported the spice from European ports to the New England states. The price of the spice commodity fluctuated due to supply and demand, thus its value dropped once the Civil War began in 1861.

The Gift of Black Pepper

When I was a child, my family was given a square wooden pepper grinder for a Christmas gift from my grandmother. It had a handle to twist for sprinkling black pepper on a pasta dish or eggs; it was so much better than fine black pepper in a can. Since then, I have discovered pepper comes in different varieties from long ago . . .

Pepper, a past treasured gift, goes back three thousand years, with roots in South India. It was not only used as a valuable spice in the spice trade. It was named "black gold" and used as currency. The pepper comes from the vine of the *Piperaceae* family; it is a fruit aka peppercorn. Pepper contains the compound piperine. During ancient days, black pepper folklore touts pepper healed many ailments, including indigestion, insomnia, joint pain, and toothaches. Fresh ground pepper is more flavorful than ground.

Baharat, an Arabic spice blend, includes black pepper, found in Mediterranean cuisine. Black pepper and black lemon pepper (made from granulated lemon zest and cracked black peppercorns) are common spices. And there are colored peppercorns, too. On a dinner menu in Toronto, Canada, I ordered Grain Salad: spinach, crispy chickpeas, watermelon, beets, strawberry peppercorn vinaigrette. These and pink, green peppercorns and white pepper are found at specialty stores.

#8 Modern North American Era: In the early twentieth century, herbs and spices continued to gain attention for their medicinal merits. Scientists around the globe isolated and studied medicinal compounds from plants for potential healing benefits. Both fresh herbs and dried herbs and spices were making a splash. Not only were they commonplace in home gardens and nurseries, but dried herbs and spices were found in supermarkets and grocery stores, big and small.

During the twenty-first century, through the growing awareness of natural health and a backlash against using pharmaceutical drugs with undesirable side effects, herbs and spices have made a great comeback. As different cultures and generations seek adventure in food, herbs and spices play a major role in offering new tastes. Not only are culinary needs met but healing benefits are of value, too. And the herb and spice industries are blossoming . . .

A SPICE GURU: THE SPICE HOUSE INNOVATOR

Let me introduce you to a pioneer in the herb and spice world, Patricia A. Erd. She is the owner of The Spice House, a family-owned business that goes back almost a half a century. Patricia considers The Spice House a special place. Her parents' original spice shop was located in Milwaukee, and more stores followed as the business flourished. But now, the Chicago store is the flagship. Here are a few questions I asked the spice wizard. Her answers are enlightening.

Q: *How many stores do you have?*
A: We have four locations. My parents moved to downtown Milwaukee forty years ago, and we have had a store on Old World Third Street ever since. Tom, my husband, and I own that building; and it has a wonderful food history, as it was a German Konditorei [the German word for a confectionary shop] back in the 1800s.

Q: *Is there more memorable history linked to your spice shops?*
A: We have some pages recorded as oral history from the daughter of the patisserie owners, and it is surprising how much the lives of those small business owners are reflective of ours. There was a note about how they were just too tired to celebrate Christmas as it was nonstop work leading up to it. In the early days, before we could afford a staff, Tom and I worked eighty-plus-hour work weeks.

Q: *Why do you feel herbs and spices are so popular now? From the millennials to boomers, it seems we're going back to nature.*
A: We have found spices and herbs to be sought after throughout most of the history of the world. In this country, their desirability has been enhanced by our knowledge of different cuisines and wanting to explore deliciousness. We stick to culinary application, but the crossover between spices being used in cooking having healing properties seems to be gaining interest.

Q: *What are your personal favorite Mediterranean herbs and spices?*
A: I love so many of our hand-mixed blends that it would be like

trying to pick a favorite child! What you are going to fall in love with depends upon what your favorite foods are to cook. Sunny Paris Seasoning is at the top of our list. It is a salt-free blend that is a tricky one to make. Its ingredients are chervil, dill weed, freeze-dried scallions, French basil, ground green peppercorns, minced parsley flakes, shallots, and tarragon. I love it on fresh fish, eggs, and all vegetables. It is versatile and we use it at home.

Q: *How have spices been a life changer for you?*

A: Over the years we have had at least five marriages among our employees who have met while working at The Spice House. Some of these have resulted in the next generation! It is a rewarding experience to love what you do, and our employees all share a common bond of the love of cooking. Life is good.

MORE PAST USES OF HERBS AND SPICES

The colorful history of herbs and spices includes many groups of people and methods of use. Below, take a glance at the users, events, and benefits reaped centuries ago. The historical observations are sourced from a consensus of food historians, herbalists, and proponents of seasonings.

User	Event	What It Did
Sumerians	Noted healing powers of herbs	Medicinal uses helped digestion
Chinese	Used hundreds of herbs	Healing powers for physical ailments
Egyptians	Used herbs and spices topically, cosmetic, and culinary	Preserving deceased, natural cleaning, adding flavor and freshness to food
Greeks	Imported spices from Asia, used herbs from Mediterranean countries	Putting the healing powers of herbs and spices to work.

| Europeans | Stocked gardens with herbs | These were sold at apothecaries for medicinal benefits |

HERBS AND SPICES MILESTONES

Certain key dates and key people have been connected to the popularity of herbs and spices. Food historians and herbalists agree about these particular happenings and the people who were gamechangers in the world of seasoning. Here is a look at some of them.

Year	What Happened	What It Did
1000 b.c.	Queen Sheba offered King Solomon spices with gold and stones	It showed that spices were believed to be valuable
2700 b.c.	Shen Nung penned *The Classic Herbal*	Provided recognition of dozens of healing plants
3rd millennium B.C.	Sumerian clay tablets noted aromatic plants	Proof of awareness of herbs
668–633 B.C.	King Ashurbanipal of Assyria recorded aromatic plants	Showed benefits of herbs and spices
721–710 B.C.	King Merodach-baladan II of Babylonia grew dozens of plants in his garden	Heightened awareness of herbs and spices harvested from plants
460–377 B.C.	Physician Hippocrates documented data about herbs and spices	He pointed out that herbs and spices provided medicinal benefits
First century	Physician Dioscorides *De Materia Midica*	Reference for usage of herbs and spices in health remedies
Ninth century	Arab doctors used herbs and spices	Herbs and spices were known for flavoring benefits

Year	What Happened	What It Did
Ninth century	Emperor Charlemagne noted several dozens of herbs	A variety of herbs were to be harvested at his royal estates and used for medicinal purposes
Sixteenth century	Christopher Columbus, Ferdinand Magellan, and Marco Polo created the momentum of finding new routes to obtain spices for Europe	Herbs and spices were used to ward off the bubonic plague during the Middle Ages
Eighteenth century	Jonathan Carnes, sea captain from Massachusetts, started spice trading	It ignited more usage of spices
Nineteenth	William M. McCormick created McCormick & Company	Distribution of spices and seasoning mixes offered to America for culinary usage
Twentieth century	Mrs. M. Grieve wrote A Modern Herbal in the 1930s	The text enlightened the mainstream audience about usage of herbs

All-Purpose Healing

Homemade Spicy Dry Rub

One Thanksgiving my S.O. cooked an all-natural turkey for us. Basted with butter and sprinkled with salt and pepper, the bird became a dull nondescript meal. Later, my male friend and I had a tiff over the trivial matter because

I noted the bird was bland. It was! To show his frustration he wrapped the rest of his fowl in foil, put it in the shotgun seat of his fancy car, and drove home. I felt relieved knowing the flavorless bird was out of sight, out of mind.

This spicy rub recipe, which comes from a popular chocolate company, dishes big flavor. The ingredients are sure to please when cooking up a bird. It will spice up any poultry or meat, feed the senses, and perhaps keep the peace in your household.

Baked chicken thighs
6 tablespoon hot cocoa mix
5 tablespoons roasted cacao nibs
5 tablespoons finely chopped almonds
1 tablespoon chipotle powder (or for less smoky flavor
*   use chili flakes)*
5 tablespoons paprika
1 tablespoon garlic powder
2 teaspoons ground cinnamon
2 teaspoons dried oregano
½ teaspoon mustard powder
2 teaspoons onion powder
5 teaspoons salt
2 teaspoons ground cumin
1 teaspoon freshly ground black pepper
1 tablespoon sumac powder
½ cup brown sugar
Pumpkin seeds, for garnish

Using a large chef's knife, finely chop almonds. Whisk all ingredients together in a bowl.

Rub surfaces of boneless chicken thighs with olive oil, then coat with spicy rub (it includes all ingredients including cocoa nibs and almonds).[Coat with oil to your personal preference. I recommend ½ to ¾ teaspoon for a 4 to 6 ounce thigh.] Let stand for 30 minutes at room temperature or refrigerate up to 8 hours. Preheat the oven to 450 degrees F and bake for 18 minutes until internal temperature of chicken is 165 degrees F. Garnish with toasted pumpkin seeds. Do not re-use rub that has been in contact with raw meat.

This spicy recipe is easy to make and worth the effort to spice up baked chicken or an outdoor barbecue... All the different spices is sure to please the palate for carnivores! Note: One chicken thigh is an average serving for one person.

Makes 2 cups. (Note: One chicken thigh is about 3 ounces of meat, so a serving can be one or two thighs per person)

(Courtesy: Lake Champlain Chocolates)

In the next part of this book, you'll discover 22 well-loved versatile herbs and spices categorized from A to Z. Folk remedies using the chosen picks combined with each other and/or some other seasonings, too, will follow later with more practical DIY ways to use herbs and spices.

HEALING HIGHLIGHTS FROM NATURE'S GARDEN-FEST

✓ Specific herbs and spices owned up to their versatility, in biblical times and the stone age, but exactly how they worked wonder was often unclear.

✓ Usage of herbs and spices goes back at least five thousand years. Aromatic plants were foraged by hunters and gatherers and put to work for flavoring and preserving food.

✓ Century by century, herbs and spices continued to gain popularity in many countries.

✓ At the end of the 1700s, America was part of the world spice trade.

✓ But in the mid-part of the 1800s, the large supply of spices generated a sharp decline and the demand for the pepper trade plummeted once the Civil War began in 1861.

✓ In the eighteenth and nineteenth centuries, scientists conducting lab studies began to pinpoint specific chemical compounds in herbs and spices. Their findings helped show how properties work in seasonings, leading to suggesting potential health advantages.

✓ Fast-forward to the twenty-first century, studies on health benefits of nature's herbs and spices are ongoing around the world.

✓ Health benefits linked to compounds in herbs and spices are publicized as nature's medicine. Herbs and spices are used as a healing aid for both conventional and holistic medicine.

PART 2

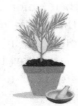

TOP 22 GARDEN GIFTS

ENTERING NATURE'S BOTANICAL GARDEN

My chosen 22 herbs and spices are treasured, by me, and people past and present-day. About 75 percent of these picks are gleaned from the Oldways Mediterranean Diet pyramid foods chart. More than half of these seasonings have roots from Mediterranean countries. Others, while not originating in Europe, made their way there by trade and demand. In time, the Mediterranean herbs and spices became popular in the United States, just like the Mediterranean diet and lifestyle.

In the pages that follow, I will introduce each herb and spice in a reader-friendly format: I share a personal story, the history of the herbs and spices, their compounds and nutrients, some studies for diseases, other health ailments, and how to use each one to enjoy the legendary healing powers. And then, a flavorful and nutritious recipe shows how you can put these herbs and spices to work—titillating your senses and boosting your health. You can find definitions of some of the essential vitamins, minerals, and compounds in the glossary.

After you get acquainted with each herb and spice, it's time to mix it up. I include the basic chosen herbs and spices and add them to blends that will rock your world and household. I share how these extraordinary taste pleasers can help you to slim down, shape up, and stall the aging process. And there's more . . .

This book contains more than forty-three home cures for common ailments, such as anxiety, colds, flu, insomnia, muscle aches, PMS, stress, and more. You'll also learn how to be delighted by each and every seasoning in Mediterranean diet recipes for all four seasons.

Allspice

(Myrtaceae)

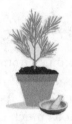

The air was full of spices.
—Frances Hodgson Burnett, *A Little Princess*

One of my favorite pastimes as a kid was playing sous chef, using my mother's kitchen stocked with baking spices—and discovering the wonder of allspice. On a rainy, fall day I found an apple muffin recipe in one of my mom's cookbooks. In the kitchen cupboard the McCormick's red and white cans marked cinnamon and nutmeg were empty. I grabbed a glass jar of allspice. It was a dark ground powder with the aroma of the MIA spices. "Maybe this will work," I thought, like a mad scientist throwing caution away in favor of the foreign ingredient, and hoped for the best.

After dinner that night I announced my baking surprise. "I made a batch of spicy apple muffins! Try one." Like a judge on a TV cooking show, my mom complimented my use of the complex flavors of my spice choice. Making her smile was like an antidepressant drug. Maybe a magical compound in the allspice lightened her serious mood, naturally. But I was just a kid. What did I know? She ate two muffins and didn't reprimand me for a flopped dessert. "They are good," she pronounced, and her words rang with conviction. "Really good. What spice did you use?"

I chuckled. "It's my secret." I felt empowered as I realized that baking is a creative venture and that sometimes you have to take a risk by trusting your instincts.

The Family Tree of Allspice

Welcome to a spice that comes from an evergreen tree growing in subtropical regions, such as South America and the West Indies. White flowers and purple berries are its hallmarks. When the berries are plucked and dried, they look much like black pepper.

Don't let the name "allspice" confuse you. Actually, it does not contain all spices. However, its aroma and flavor are similar to those of cloves, cinnamon, ginger, and nutmeg. Allspice was used five hundred years ago and grew in popularity once the explorer Columbus introduced it to Europe. It was used for a variety of foods, since it can be paired easily with both savory and sweet dishes.

Caribbean people used allspice as a natural cure-all for a variety of ailments, from stomach woes to the common cold. It is believed the Mayan Indians used allspice for embalming the deceased. In Europe, it was used for superstitious reasons, such as bringing riches. Allspice also has roots in the cuisine of the Mediterranean world where it is used for flavoring fish, eggs, cheese, breads, and desserts likes cakes and cookies.

Columbus and His Peppery Accidental Discovery

Christopher Columbus set sail in search of spices. He carried peppercorns with him on his 1493 voyage to the New World so that when he made landfall, the local nature-oriented scientists could tell him where to find pepper.

The natives in the Caribbean told the explorer that the berries grew wild on the islands. It turned out the island berries were allspice—not pepper. But Columbus didn't have a naturalist with him, so he believed what he was told. After all, allspice berries look like big peppercorns, which come from an evergreen, not a plant—another reason why allspice berries could be mistaken for peppercorns. Allspice became known as pimento, a link to the Spanish word for pepper.[1]

On his fourth voyage, when he landed in Jamaica, Columbus discovered allspice. Alas, he dubbed the spice "Jamaican pepper." Once he brought the berries to Europe, when the English people tasted his peppered spice, they coined it "allspice" because of its flavor of cinnamon, cloves, ginger, and nutmeg. Despite the adventurer's faux pas in misnaming the amazing allspice, his efforts have been remembered.

Allspice Plant Power: Surprise Stuff

Allspice is an amazing gift of nature, chock-full of chemical compounds and nutrients. Eugenol, an anti-inflammatory compound (inflammation is the root of many ailments and diseases), makes up 75 percent of the ingredients in allspice. But it doesn't stop there.

Cineole, another anti-inflammatory and antioxidant; quercetin, another antioxidant; myrcene, a brain chemical booster; and phellandrene, an antibacterial are just some of the components that make allspice all it can be. Allspice also includes limonene—another antioxidant and anti-inflammatory compound that all together make this spice intriguing to scientists who study its health-giving benefits.

Its nutrients include vitamins A, C, the antioxidant beta carotene, and the B vitamins. Its minerals include copper, iron, magnesium, manganese, and another antioxidant selenium. With a good-for-you essential nutrients line up like this, allspice is all you would need if you had to choose just one spice.

GROUNDBREAKING DISCOVERIES

Since allspice contains disease-fighting antioxidants, can it help lower the risk of developing heart disease? Perhaps. After all this ancient spice contains phytochemicals that help to keep you heart-healthy, especially paired with low-fat, nutrient dense foods and when its flavor makes us less inclined to overuse salt.

Allspice may even help guard against cancer. Research published in the journal *Carcinogenesis* suggests that allspice and its compounds ericifolin may help protect men from developing prostate cancer. Evidently, the so-called chemotherapeutic agents come from nature's plants, including spices like allspice. It was discovered that ericifolin may "silence" cancer-causing cells and inhibit growth of cancer. It will take more research to confirm that eating allspice can guard against cancer, but adding a natural spice, like this, shows promise and may be of benefit when added to a low-fat, nutrient-rich diet.[2]

Bountiful Benefits: Allspice may help improve asthma symptoms, blood circulation, and help heal wounds. As a folk remedy, allspice is helpful for digestive complaints, from stomachache to a detoxifying remedy. Thanks to its anti-inflammatory compounds, allspice may help to lessen aches and pains. If you're trying to lose unwanted pounds, allspice may even be one of the go-to weight loss spices. (Refer to the chapter "Season Up, Slim Down.")

Spice It Up Now! Allspice is ideal for baking spicy cakes, cookies, muffins, and pies, especially apple pastries during the fall. And it is also good for cooking! Folklore accounts say allspice may bring good luck and fortune. On New Year's Day I bake a batch of round (the shape symbolizes money), spicy Snickerdoodles and add allspice for good luck. Allspice berries store well and you can grind them into powder or purchase the ready-made ground powder variety for convenience. I also use allspice to spice up fish—with the aroma and flavor of the combo powerhouse of spices it's ideal.

Heart-Healthy

Allspice Apple Muffins

Autumn, swimming, and spicy muffins are three of my favorite things. One late fall, I chose to swim in a hotel's outdoor pool during a snowstorm. The water was warm with its steam rising into the freezing air, but getting out was a challenge. I cherish the memory of ordering a large spicy apple muffin with raw sugar on top after my swim. Since you know I've mastered the art of baking apple muffins as a kid, I will now share my recipe.

2½ cups cake flour
½ cup golden brown sugar
¼ cup white granulated sugar
1 teaspoon allspice (Mountain Rose Herbs)
½ teaspoon cinnamon
4 large brown eggs
1 cup European-style butter, melted
2 teaspoons orange extra virgin olive oil
2 cups Granny Smith and Honeycrisp apples, cored,
    peeled, chopped
1 teaspoon pure vanilla
½ cup hazelnuts or pecans
¼ cup (each) pecans and almonds
Mediterranean sea salt to taste
Cinnamon-sugar (McCormick)

Preheat the oven to 400 degrees F. In a bowl, measure the flour, sugar, and spices. Set aside. In a separate bowl, whisk together the eggs, butter, and oil until blended. Fold in apples and add vanilla. Pour this mixture over the dry ingredients and mix. Stir in nuts. Spoon the batter evenly into a muffin tin. Use the rest of the batter in a small-size bread pan (unless you want larger-size muffins) and lightly grease with orange olive oil. Yes, it works. Drop nuts on top of muffins (and bread). Bake for about 20 minutes (it takes a bit longer in higher altitude) till the surface turns a firm golden brown (or until a knife inserted into the center of the muffin comes out clean). Sprinkle with cinnamon-sugar or sea salt on top of muffins.

The fresh baked spicy and sweet apples will fill your home with tantalizing aromas. These warm and moist creations, sweetened with the chunks of apples, are something to write home about. The crunch of the mixed nuts and saltiness of Mediterranean sea salt (like the spice used on gourmet dark chocolate caramels) this time around is also a perfect Italian-style combo. If you don't want to overindulge—pop some muffins into the freezer.

Makes 12 medium-size muffins and one small-size bread.

As you can see, allspice is a fascinating spice that belongs in your spice rack year-round—not just during autumn and the holiday season. There is another super spice that is making a comeback. It is good to stock and savor for all seasons. Go ahead—discover the world of anise in the next chapter.

HEALING HIGHLIGHTS FROM NATURE'S GARDEN-FEST

✓ Aromatic allspice boosts flavors in both savory and sweet foods because it contains a combination of spices.

✓ Don't be fooled as Christopher Columbus was . . . The Italian explorer discovered allspice, but he thought it was the super find of pepper, most likely because the pepper berries resemble peppercorns.

✓ Allspice contains anti-inflammatory components that may lessen pain, naturally—without the side effects of pain-relieving drugs.

✓ The four-in-one spice can also aid other health ailments, from

the common cold to a stomachache. Your symptoms may go
AWOL after putting allspice to work. (Refer to the herbal healings chapter.)

✓ allspice roots are Caribbean, but its healing powers are universal.

✓ It's a multipurpose spice providing heart-healthy benefits, and
even better when used with a Mediterranean diet—for both baking and cooking.

✓ Some folks use allspice to boost brainpower and add it in a cup of
tea or coffee. Wakey wakey!

✓ And note, using one spice instead of many spices can be easier on
the pocketbook and a convenient substitute in case you don't
have access to a spice you need.

Anise

(Umbellifarae)

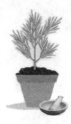

*Woe unto you, scribes and Pharisees, hypocrites! for
ye pay tithe of mint and anise and cummin, and have
omitted the weightier matters of the law, judgment,
mercy, and faith: these ought ye to have done, and not
to leave the other undone.*
—MATTHEW 23:23, *New Testament*

On a Sunday night one winter in my childhood years, a special guest
arrived at the front door for after-dinner coffee and anise cookies. We
served the fresh spice cookies to the imperial-like priest sitting on our
sofa. He was the man who preached dramatic soap opera–type ser-
mons every Sunday morning. I watched him dip the Italian cookies
into espresso coffee. And soon, the tall elderly Italian cleric clad in a
Roman collar around his neck with street clothes appeared relaxed.

He smiled and laughed while nibbling the cookies that smelled like licorice.

I gave credit to the cookies that helped our guest feel calmer. But what did I know? I was just a nosy kid playing with my Dalmatian. I listened to the priest share a story about his first canine in Tuscany when he was a boy. On that evening I had an epiphany: Our chief priest was not royalty or a saint. He was a down-to-earth man who liked cookies and dogs, as well as a fine orator. In hindsight, I believe an ingredient in the anise uplifted his mindful manner and let him feel at ease in our home.

THE FAMILY TREE OF ANISE

Anise is one of the spices noted in the Bible as a healing food. Like pepper, anise was used as payment, which shows how valuable it was to people. Historians tell us the anise seed was originally grown in the Mediterranean regions and Egypt. It is believed that ancient Egyptians used anise to quell aches and pains, such as a toothache.

As time passed, anise was imported to Mediterranean countries and grown there. Then, the word spread about its healing powers and anise got acknowledgment around the globe. It may have started as a flavoring agent for entrées and desserts, but its versatility and healing powers don't stop there.

ANISE PLANT POWER: SURPRISE STUFF

The chemical compound dubbed "anethole" is what provides that sweet, licorice taste to anise seed. Other constituents in anise consist of acetophenone, anethole, anise alcohol, estragole, limonene, p-anisaldehyde, and pinene. The active components are so potent that anise was included in medicine provided to fight strong strains of flu, like the Swine Flu back in 2009.

Not only does anise boast healing chemical compounds, it also contains a whopping amount of nutrients, too. One tablespoon of anise seed can add iron, bone-boosting manganese, and calcium to your diet. These three minerals are important for women and every bit helps. It also contains 1 gram of protein and 0.9 grams of dietary fiber.

Of course, you would not consume almost one-half cup of anise, but the following chart, which uses a common measurement, gives you an idea of its impressive nutritional value.

ANISE SEEDS

Nutrition facts for a serving size containing 100 grams (31/2 ounces):

	Nutrient Value	Percentage of RDA
Calories	337	17
Carbohydrates	50.02 g	38
Protein	17.60 g	31
Cholesterol	0 mg	0
Dietary fiber	14.6 g	38
Vitamins		
Niacin	3.060 mg	19
Pantothenic acid	0.797 mg	16
Pyridoxine	0.650 mg	50
Riboflavin	0.290 mg	22
Thiamin	0.340 mg	28
Vitamin A	311 IU	10.5
Vitamin C	31 mg	35
Sodium	16 mg	1
Potassium	1,441 mg	31

Minerals

Calcium	646 mg	65
Magnesium	170 mg	42.5
Manganese	2,300 mg	100
Phosphorus	440 mg	63
Selenium	5.0 mg	9
Zinc	5.30 mg	48

(Source: USDA Nutrient Database)

Star Anise, a Stunning Spice

Let me introduce this Chinese spice that comes from the dried star-shaped fruit grown on an evergreen tree. This brown-colored star anise resembles starfish in the sea. Historical healing powers include "Chinese herbalists using star anise as a stimulant, an expectorant, and digestion aid," as stated by the Herb Society of America (HSA). "Also, European healers used it for teas for rheumatism and chewing the seed for indigestion."

Moreover, this spice contains "shikimic acid which is one of the primary components of the influenza-fighting drug Tamiflu," adds the HSA. Research suggests extracts from star anise contain antifungal and antimicrobial compounds. Star anise also contains some of the components of anise seeds, with its distinctive licorice aroma and flavor. So it can be used in baking—but it must be ground and not left intact despite its beauty. I have noticed it is used as a garnish (not to be eaten) to beautify the presentation of baked goods, often during autumn and winter holidays.

Spiced Star Anise Hot Chocolate

Oregon-based Mountain Rose Herbs' customers have said that they enjoy this exotic spice in broths and spice blends, which includes Chinese Five-Spice Blend and Five Spice Powder. One of the company's office sweet and spicy favorites is using star anise in a reishi hot chocolate. (Reishi slices are herbal mushrooms also used in tea.)

2 ounces organic whole cacao beans
5 organic whole bird's eye chilis
4 organic sweet cinnamon sticks
2 organic whole star anise pods
4 cups milk (or your favorite alternative)
6 organic reishi slices (Mountain Rose Herbs)
1 tablespoon organic vanilla powder
½ teaspoon organic nutmeg powder
Large tea ball infuser, 4-inch tea net or cheesecloth

Break cacao beans in half and rub between your palms to create cacao nibs and hulls. Add cacao nibs and hulls, chilis, cinnamon sticks, and star anise to tea infuser or cheesecloth bundle. Add milk, reishi slices, tea infuser, vanilla powder, and nutmeg powder to a medium pot. Bring to a boil, then reduce heat to low and cover. Let gently simmer for 30 minutes. Strain tea infuser and remove reishi slices. Ladle into your favorite mug and serve immediately.

Makes 3 large cups.

*Author's note: I tweaked the recipe for my taste. I used low-fat organic milk, left out reishi slices, and substituted vanilla powder with ½ teaspoon pure vanilla extract.

(Courtesy: Mountain Rose Herbs)

GROUNDBREAKING DISCOVERIES

Anise isn't just for baking. It's got medicinal powers that may be of interest to you or someone you know. This ancient spice is believed to be of use to help lessen depression. Popping an antidepressant pill is often prescribed by a doctor, but the anise remedy may work to boost out-of-sync chemicals in the brain, too.

Past research has shown some improvement among people suffering from irritable bowel syndrome, who had less depression when given anise oil (which is extracted from the plant). More research is needed because scientists don't agree on exactly how the spice works.[1]

Another study published in the *Journal of Research in Medical Sciences* showed anise may have real antidepressant virtues. That's the word from Iranian researchers, who say anise compounds in anise seeds helped relieve symptoms of postpartum depression. But note, the jury is still out on pinpointing the exact properties in anise seeds that lessen depression. The anethole compound may boost serotonin (a brain chemical that can make you feel happier and enhance brain power and memory.[2]

Blessed with its multitude of components, its anethole found in the oil of anise is believed to be a good thing for blood circulation. During our youthful days, we don't think about heart and strokes. But as we age, since the anethole may lessen the formation of blood clots—it seems like it's spice for thought.

Bountiful Benefits: Anise is also used to ease the hacking cough that is common with seasonal allergies or after coping with a common cold. As a kid, I recall enjoying licorice-flavored cough drops to soothe a sore throat. Jakeman's throat and chest lozenges, originated in 1907, were flavored with anise. More recently, I can attest to anise's ability to soothe my spring symptoms brought on by drifting pollen and a shedding pooch.

Safety Sound Bite: Pregnant women should stay clear of consuming anise because of its anethole, which may induce premature labor.

Shake It Up Now! Both anise seeds and leaves can be used for flavor and healthful benefits. This licorice-flavored spice is often used in entrée dishes such as soups and baked goods like biscotti. I have used

McCormick's anise extract in baking cookies. It isn't uncommon to find anise-flavored coffee (I tried it during the holidays) or you can brew the seeds in hot water, strain it, and enjoy the spice in a cup of tea. Anise can also be found in essential oils, and both bar and liquid soaps. Star anise is so pretty it's no surprise it is used in crafts, such as a homemade wreath or potpourri.

Mood Enhancing
Jumbo Anise Biscotti

❖ ❖ ❖

I love biscotti. Baking up a batch isn't too difficult, but it does take some time and a skill set to make the cookies uniform in their oblong shapes. Before a book event I begged my dear friend Gemma Sciabica to bake biscotti for the audience. She obliged. I lacked confidence in baking these Italian cookies. The secret is, don't focus on making the twice-baked cookies perfectly uniform in shape and size. Once you move away from that line of thinking, it's actually quite easy to do. Since biscotti often has an anise flavor, why not use homemade cookies to dip into a cup of tea or Italian roast? This recipe is inspired by all the strong women mentors in my life.

¾ cup almonds chopped coarsely
3 eggs (or 6 egg whites)
5 tablespoons Marsala Olive Fruit Oil
2 tablespoons Galliano or Strega
1 tablespoon anise seeds
¼ teaspoon anise extract
1 teaspoon vanilla
Grated peel of 1 orange or 1 lemon
2½ cups flour
1¼ teaspoons baking powder
1 teaspoon salt
1 cup sugar

Preheat the oven to 350 degrees F. Place almonds in small baking pan. Toast until light golden, about 10 minutes, cool, chop coarsely. Grease large cookie sheet. In a small bowl add eggs, olive oil, and flavorings. In another bowl add dry ingredients, flour, baking powder, salt, and sugar. Make well in the center. Pour egg mixture into flour mixture, stir until dough holds together. Place dough on floured surface, knead until just well blended. Cut dough in half. With floured fingers, shape the dough into logs about 10 inches by 3 inches. Bake for 25 minutes or until firm to the touch and light golden brown. Remove from oven, let cool about 15 minutes. With serrated knife cut each log straight or diagonally into 1-inch- or 1¼-inch-thick slices. Place biscotti back on cookie sheet, bake about 10 minutes. Turn slices over, bake another 10 minutes to toast or until light golden brown and cookies are dry.

Makes 20 to 25.

(Courtesy: Gemma Sanita Sciabica, *Baking with California Olive Oil: Dolci and Biscotti Recipes*)

Let's move onward to the tree with a mystical history—and gives us magical leaves. It's time to meet the aromatic bay leaf.

HEALING HIGHLIGHTS FROM NATURE'S GARDEN-FEST

✓ Cheer up! Healing compounds like anethole in anise can act as a mood booster, uplifting your spirit . . .
✓ Did you know the anise seed is part of the parsley family of botanical plants?
✓ And do make note the anethole compound in anise may improve blood circulation, which can help enhance S-E-X.
✓ The anti-inflammatory phenylpropanoid in anise may help stave off plaque—the stuff that clogs the arteries.

✓ Coping with unsteady blood sugar levels? Adding anise seeds in a fiber-rich vegetable dish may help to get those numbers on even keel.

✓ This licorice-flavored spice is touted as a digestive aid and used in teas—DIY or store-bought.

✓ Anise isn't just for biscotti and scones—check out the aromatherapy department and European cookbooks for its versatile uses.

✓ If you're looking for that rich, enticing smell and flavor, use a small herb grinder before incorporating the spice in your food.

Bay Leaf

(Lauraceae)

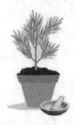

*The Bay leaves are of as necessary use as any other in
the garden or orchard, for they serve both for pleasure
and profit, both for ornament, and for use, both for
honest civil uses and for physic, yea both for the sick
and the sound, both for the living and the dead; . .*
—PARKINSON, *Garden of Flowers* (1629)

One summer afternoon, the herbal aroma in my gastronomic-ish aunt
and uncle's kitchen was a scent to cherish. As an inquisitive kid, I
stood on my tippy toes to see what was cooking in the large pot on the
stovetop. The two environmentalists who maintained a sustainable
vegetable garden were making a vegetable stew and rice dish. I studied
two leaves floating in the thick sauce.

"What are these strange things floating on top?" I asked. "California bay leaves," the schoolteachers answered in unison. I scrutinized the wilted leaves like a foreign spider on the floor. "Do we have to eat these?" I questioned, recalling the yucky gourmet stew dishes my mom made that I refused to try. "I'll toss the leaves when the stew is done," my aunt said, laughing. There was a collective sigh of relief between me and my younger brother who preferred no-frills food with our unsophisticated palates. Whenever I smell the earth aroma of bay leaves, it takes me back to my childhood, on that day I had a flavorful dish with a bay leaf taste.

Years later I lived in the Santa Cruz Mountains, a place where laurel trees grow. I often make a vegetarian stew full of aroma and flavor, inspired by my aunt and uncle's recipes. And nowadays, for memory's sake, a jar of bay leaves sits on the wooden round spice rack on a shelf in the cupboard, like my herb-smart relatives had in their breathtaking pantry.

THE FAMILY TREE OF BAY LEAF

The pungent, minty fragrant dried bay laurel is a timeless herb linked to "wisdom" that goes back centuries. Bay leaf comes from an evergreen tree known as the *Laurus nobilis*. It grows in the Mediterranean region and even Mendocino, Northern California, a town with a natural vibe that I've visited. The beautiful laurel tree, like eucalyptus in Monterey, can grow more than two dozen feet, with telltale light-colored flowers and blackberries. The leaves were called "bay" back in ancient days and were popular with both Greeks and Romans. Herb history enthusiasts will tell you that the Greeks created bay leaf crowns for athletes and heroes to wear.

The bay leaf was touted for its healing powers throughout the centuries. Native Americans used their herb in a salve mixed with other herbs to prevent seizures. It is believed some tribes inhaled the bay leaf as a headache remedy. It was used during the Middle Ages, especially to help lower the risk of catching the deadly bubonic plague. As an aromatic and savory herb, it fared well in both medicinal uses and culinary delights.

The Legend of Apollo, Love, and the Bay Tree

As the bittersweet Greek myth goes, Daphne, a beautiful and free-spirited woman, was admired by Apollo, the Greek god of sun and light. Instead of becoming an object of Apollo's desire, she pleaded with her father, the river god Ladonas, to transform her. He granted Daphne her wish. The end result? She was morphed into an independent stunning, lean bay laurel tree—and Apollo was left without Daphne, his human love interest.

Another version of the legend claims Apollo was struck by Cupid's arrow. He pursued Daphne but his love was unrequited. So Apollo, still smitten by the lady, transformed her into bay laurel, whom he cherished. He claimed the beautiful tree to be his own and deemed it an accomplishment.

BAY LEAF PLANT POWER: SURPRISE STUFF

There are a variety of types of bay leaves but it's the Turkish that is the most popular. Others include California, Indian, Indonesian, and sweet. The bay leaf, whatever type, is a powerful plant with powerful compounds. Yes, that strange-looking, savory and potent bay leaf used in hearty soups and stews that I loved as a young'un and still adore in fall and winter months is a superherb!

Let me introduce 1,8-cineole, also named "eucalyptol," which is found in eucalyptus oil. This compound makes up about 75 percent of the herb. It is praised for its antibacterial, anti-inflammatory, and anti-fungal healing powers. Some properties in bay leaf include anti–bug repellent lauric acid and parthenolides, which research shows can help provide relief for headaches.

The bay leaf is modest in its nutritional box. The first fact that caught my attention is that it's low calorie: One tablespoon contains a mere five calories. The leaf does have modest amounts of iron and vitamin A. But truly, you get more of these nutrients in apricots. The fact remains, it's the antioxidant value paired with nutritious foods that's going to give you the healing power boost.

GROUNDBREAKING DISCOVERIES

Past research hints that bay leaf extracts may help to cause breast cancer cells to die. Also, colorectal cancer may also benefit from bay leaf because it stalls cancer cells from growing. Eucalyptol, the immune-enhancing chemical compound, may actually be helpful in lowering the risk of developing cancers, like these. More research is needed but for now including bay leaf in a nutritious Mediterranean diet and lifestyle may be worth the effort.

So, can foraging California bay leaf help fight cancer? Probably not. But if you include antioxidant-rich bay leaf in a nutrient-rich daily diet and get a move on (whether it's hiking to find the laurel tree or walking the dog), the exercise may help boost your cardiovascular health and immune system, too.

Bay leaf may also be just what the doctor should order to stave off type 2 diabetes. Past research shows it may lower high sugar levels, cholesterol, and triglycerides. Credit is given to its multitude of compounds—not just one. The positive effects on people, though, are not definitive. Bay leaves (no specific variety) have been shown to improve insulin function (in test-tube experiments) and show potential. Meanwhile, more studies are needed to prove it can indeed be the anti-diabetes prescription instead of taking medications.[1]

Bountiful Benefits: Bay leaf may help enhance digestion, including uncomfortable flatulence and bloating. It also is known to lessen aches and pain in muscles and joints. The hardy leaves provide folk remedies for dry scalp to skin problems. And some folk remedy proponents tout its healing powers in wound recovery and in helping people coping with blood sugar ups and downs.

Shake It Up Now! Bay leaves are used for aromatherapy, since bay leaf can be a delightful and uplifting fragrance, especially as an essential oil. Bay leaf is also used as incense for the home. The distinct bay leaf is included in body fragrances, cosmetics, and cleansers, such as a natural bay leaf soap bar for women and men.

Bay leaf, which is known to grow in Northern California and up to the West Coast, is praised for its down-to-earth flavor used in cooking a variety of Mediterranean dishes. Bay leaves are found dried at supermarkets (California and Turkish varieties are available online). If you want to use Indian Bay visit an Indian specialty market. Once eliminated, the flavor and aroma linger leaving its pungent telltale herbal essence.

Safety Sound Bite: Toss the bay leaf after using it in a cooked dish. It's too tough with rugged edges and should not be eaten.

Antioxidant-Rich, Disease-Fighting

Mussels Marinara Sauce with Bay Leaf and Rice

Shellfish and pasta: two foods that transcend me to memorable dinners overlooking the water on Fisherman's Wharf in San Francisco. Growing up in the San Francisco Bay Area and going to college in the city, I often enjoyed shellfish dishes with friends, family, and past loves. This recipe is inspired by home, close to my heart and memories throughout decades of visiting the dock of the bay.

Macaroni and cheese in a box to canned SpaghettiOs were my favorite pasta dishes when I was a tween. Then, Fettucine with Fresh Tomatoes and Basil, Pasta Primavera, and shellfish and pasta plates entered my life. This recipe is a good one, especially if you're a carnivore, so instead of giving you a fish version (I have substituted crab for sausage), here is the real deal.

4 dozen mussels, cleaned well (or clams)
½ pound Italian sausage, cooked, sliced thin
⅓ cup Marsala Olive Fruit Oil
1 onion, chopped
4 garlic cloves, chopped
1 leek (white part only), chopped
1 bell pepper, diced
4 tomatoes, chopped

½ cup fresh parsley, chopped
1 cup white wine
2 bay leaves
Salt, pepper, and cayenne to taste
4 slices crusty Italian bread, toasted
3 to 4 tablespoons tomato paste

Rinse mussels thoroughly in cold running water, scrub, pull off beard. Cover with water for 1 hour, discard mussels that float to the top or are opened. Cook sausage with 1 cup water until browned. Lift out with slotted spoon, drain on clean paper towel. In Dutch oven add oil, onion, garlic, leek, and pepper, cook until crisp tender. Add tomatoes, parsley, wine, bay leaves, salt, pepper, and cayenne, bring to boil. Add mussels, cook covered 5 to 8 minutes. Stir in cooked sausage. Discard any unopened mussels, remove bay leaves. Place bread in soup bowls, place mussels and cooking liquid atop. Mussels may be served over cooked pasta, polenta or rice. Add 3 to 4 tablespoon of tomato paste in liquid, cook about 10 minutes. Add a little more wine if needed.

Serves 4.

(Courtesy: Gemma Sanita Sciabica, *Cooking with California Olive Oil: Treasured Family Recipes*)

Now that bay leaf is in your spice cabinet, it's time to move on to an ancient Mediterranean herb and spice. Caraway seeds are surprisingly little wonders, too. Find out how this next herb and its healing benefits come with amazing wow factor.

HEALING HIGHLIGHTS FROM NATURE'S GARDEN-FEST

✓ Bay leaf has a history of healing powers, which the Greeks and Romans put to use in many ways.
✓ The nutrients in bay leaves are minor players, but its major play-

ers like 1,8 cineole boast big antioxidant power, making bay leaves help lower the risk of developing some diseases.

✓ Pair bay leaf in nutrient-dense, plant-based sauces and soups because it does contain heart-healthy compounds that may lower artery-clogging cholesterol even after you remove it from a dish!

✓ Do note, bay leaves are not just for cooking—even though your main course of a meal will be the best tasting EVER.

✓ Consider using bay leaf–infused personal hygiene natural products to discover how the fragrant herb can be used topically for body love!

✓ Did you know West Coast California bay taste as good as bay laurel? You can dry fresh bay leaves by putting them on a plate until dry; store them in a glass container and cool, dark cupboard.

✓ Feng shui for the New Year is healthy for the mind and body—and bay leaves used for table centers symbolizes abundance.

Caraway

(Umbelliferae)

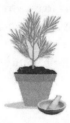

"... ta pippin and a dish of caraways"
—WILLIAM SHAKESPEARE, *Henry IV*

As a kid, it wasn't uncommon for my mom to bring home cheeses, meats, and breads for dinner. If the temperature was 100 degrees F, as it was during the dog days in San Jose, it was a no-cook meal.

One night I reached for the strange-looking oval-sliced dark rye bread. "What are these seeds?" I asked. My mom answered, "Caraway. It's the bread used for a Reuben sandwich like I ate at a café in France." While building my sandwich my mother showed me to layer pastrami, Swiss cheese, and sauerkraut with mustard and pickles. The taste of all the flavors, including the earthy caraway seeds, was far more exciting than what plain white bread could offer. I liked it. It made me feel grown up, going out of my comfort zone of white bread and trying something new.

THE FAMILY TREE OF CARAWAY

Caraway, an herb-spice, goes back to the Middle Ages in Europe. It is said the leaves of the plant are thin and with small white flowers on the tips. It's the seeds that are most flavorful and for that reason often eaten. The caraway plant's roots also go back to Asia and Africa. Historical sources show the word "caraway" goes back to the mid-fifteenth century and may have a connection to Arabia.

Caraway seeds are popular around the globe. In the Middle East it's added to desserts, in Serbia it's used in cheeses and scones—and in northern Europe, the spice is utilized in rye bread. Caraway seeds were also used in the Irish soda bread we would eat on Saint Patrick's Day and in those long breadsticks we enjoyed with homemade spicy chili.

Folklore stories include the value of caraway seeds for their uncanny ability to keep children calm. It is believed that during lengthy church services parents gave their youngsters caraway seeds to chew. Evidently, the herb help calm them. The seeds called "meetin' seeds," according to some herbalists, claim they included dill and fennel. The seeds were supposed to stave off hunger and boredom so children wouldn't disturb church services.

CARAWAY PLANT POWER: SURPRISE STUFF

The healing compound found in caraway are carvones and caveolins, which give the seed their inviting aroma and taste. And these compounds are what provide the herb with its antioxidant disease-fighting super healing powers.

Caraway seeds contain plenty of dietary fiber, since a 100-gram serving provides more than one-third of the recommended daily amount needed. Essential vitamins such as vitamins A, C, and E plus many of the good for you B vitamins are found in the little caraway seed that has big powers. Oh, and caraway boasts a bonanza of minerals, including bone-boosting calcium, energizing iron, calming magnesium, and sodium balancing, heart-healthy potassium. Speaking of heart health . . .

GROUNDBREAKING DISCOVERIES

It's no secret that dietary fiber foods, which include caraway seeds, can help keep your cholesterol at a healthy level. This, in turn, means maintaining unclogged arteries and lowering your risk of developing a heart attack or stroke. Let me explain. So, we know caraway seeds are fiber-rich. I learned years ago that fiber can lower LDL cholesterol levels (the "bad" stuff) in the body. By getting your LDL cholesterol numbers down, like we do by losing weight, exercising, eating whole grains—and caraway seeds (in moderation)—it may help reduce your risk of developing heart disease.

What's more, because caraway seeds are also rich in disease-fighting antioxidants, it can't hurt to add them to a heart-healthy Mediterranean diet. With the dietary fiber and antioxidants in caraway, you have a spice to love for life. Past research suggests caraway may be heart-healthy, but there has yet to be a sure-fire scientific study with definitive findings released. However, it couldn't hurt to add caraway seeds to your diet because of their antioxidants and nutrients.

Bountiful Benefits: Caraway is a good digestive remedy that goes way back in time when it was used as a folk remedy. Also, thanks to the relaxing mineral magnesium in caraway, if you indulge in a caraway toasted bagel or a cup of a caraway beverage, you may find yourself getting more shut-eye. And women coping with painful pre-menstrual syndromes can find relief from painful cramps by using caraway, which can soothe the nervous system. Not to forget its potential to help you to dump unwanted pounds and body fat. (See the chapter, "Season Up, Slim Down.")

Caraway, similar to anise, dill, and fennel, contains some of the same compounds. That means, it is used for its antiseptic, antispasmodic benefits as well as being a helpful digestive aid.

Shake It Up Now! Caraway seeds are used in European baking. A lot. Think of a variety of breads, breadsticks to even a British seed cake. Cooking with caraway? Why not? Caraway seeds can flavor up soups, sauces, meats, and vegetables. This herb is also used in cheese (ah, a cheese ball during the holiday season would be lovely) and salads (fruit and vegetable varieties).

As a grown-up, when I traveled to Victoria, British Columbia, appetizers were served in the hotel concierge dining room. These appetizers included caraway seed crackers and cheese (which I took back to my room with a view of the boat harbor). It was an herbal nostalgic treat, making me, the kid once timid of change, feel right at home in a foreign country. You can steep seeds in water and brew a cup of tea. Its essential oils are extracted and used in liqueurs and medications, too. Whole seeds are available at the supermarket and online.

Cholesterol-Friendly

Caraway Bread Sticks

Soup and bread sticks are part of my fondest childhood memories. On weekends in the winter, homemade vegetable soup with caraway bread sticks were served at lunch. One Sunday afternoon, I remember enjoying this hearty, hot meal in the den. My dad built a fire and we watched movies on the television. Munching on leftover caraway bread sticks and sipping hot cocoa after the soup was gone completed the comfort food day that created a lingering feeling of home and family.

1 package dry yeast
1 cup water (110 degrees F)
1 tablespoon sugar or honey
3¼ cups flour
¼ cup Marsala Olive Fruit Oil
¾ teaspoon salt (or to taste)
2 egg whites (divided)
⅓ cup caraway seeds (for top)

In a mixing bowl add yeast, water, and sugar; let stand about 10 minutes. Add remaining ingredients, flour, olive oil, salt, and 1 egg white. Stir until dough holds together.

Turn out onto lightly floured board, knead until smooth. Oil mixing bowl, place dough in, turning to coat. Cover, put in warm place to rise until doubled in bulk, about 1 hour. Turn dough out onto lightly floured board. Pat dough down to about 14 inches by 14 inches. Cut into 20 strips, roll and stretch to 12 or 14 inches long. Arrange sticks on lightly greased baking pans placed 1 inch apart. Brush with the other egg white, slightly beaten, sprinkle with caraway seeds. Let rest covered until puffy, about 20 minutes. Bake in a preheated 375-degree-F oven for 15 to 20 minutes or until golden brown.

Makes 20 to 30.

(Courtesy: Gemma Sanita Sciabica, *Cooking with California Olive Oil: Treasured Family Recipes*)

As promised, I've introduced you to some of my favorite Mediterranean herbs and spices. Cardamom, my next pick, has roots from India but it's used by many cultures and complements European foods. And yes, I, and you too, can use it in both savory and sweet dishes—not just Indian foods. Its well-rounded virtues are worth getting acquainted with. Let me introduce you to the superspice!

HEALING HIGHLIGHTS FROM NATURE'S GARDEN-FEST

✓ Caraway is a winner among many cultures, including Canada and Europe, two regions where this herb is well-loved for many reasons.

✓ One of the nutrients in caraway that I've discussed is dietary fiber, which is essential for us. It keeps us regular, which in turn provides more physical energy . . .

✓ . . . And note, this get-up-and-go vibe can increase the desire to exercise and that boosts your body's feel-good endorphins.

✓ Caraway is used in different cuisines around the world, most often in breads and cheeses—two staples in the Mediterranean diet (consumed in moderation) . . .

✓ ...And the dietary fiber in caraway seeds, when in concert with fiber-rich fruits and vegetables in the Mediterranean diet, also provides extra protection for lowering bad cholesterol, increasing good heart health.

✓ Don't forget there's more to caraway seed than breadsticks... steep them in hot water, drain, and enjoy sipping the tea while basking in the moment, being more mindful at work, play, and co-cooning at home.

✓ And remember, caraway may calm your nerves and can help you feel cool and composed—even desire to unplug.

Cardamom

(Zingiberaceae)

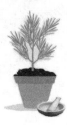

*He had prepared a pomegranate-seed dish, preserved in
almonds and sweet julep and flavored with cardamom
and rosewater, and the food was ready to serve.*
—UNKNOWN, *The Arabian Nights*

My first introduction to the citrusy-flavored spice cardamom was
when I was seventeen, dating my first love. He was born in India. It
was a tie of discovering different cultures and cuisines. One night for
my birthday he took me out to an Indian restaurant. I recall getting a
lesson on Indian food. The book-worm-ish type but sophisticated
young man, eighteen going on twenty-eight, explained how spices,
like cardamom, played a role in his food at home.

"People in my country believe cardamom tea is an aphrodisiac," he
told me once while we shared a spicy chicken dish with pita bread. For
dessert, we ordered kheer, a flowery-smelling Indian rice pudding,

which also includes cardamom smoky notes. My date grabbed a few cardamom pods piled in a dish by the cash register. "It freshens the breath," he explained, "like your candy mints."

Once inside his Volkswagen (a small, popular car in the seventies), I received my first kiss with hints of cardamom. While the jury is still out on proving whether or not cardamom is a libido enhancer, to this day I give credit to the spice for that unforgettable night. The aromatic green pods are kept inside my kitchen cupboard, which may one day give my lackluster love life a surprise nudge or two.

THE FAMILY TREE OF CARDAMOM

The spice cardamom is noted in the Bible. As we've learned its roots are traced back to India and Guatemala, too. Cardamom was a favorite used in both food and as a medicinal spice by the ancient Greeks and Romans in the Middle Ages.

As time passed, the spice was exported to different Mediterranean countries by the 1600s, thanks to sea explorers and the age of discovery. Traders from India helped create a fan base for the spice, and cardamom became commonplace in different European countries.

This spice, not unlike the herb bay leaf, was used in food and for medicinal powers, too. Interestingly, in *The Canterbury Tales* (a collection of stories by Geoffrey Chaucer, penned in Middle English, a must-read in English literature), cardamom was called "the spice of paradise."

Cardamom did also make its way to cuisine enjoyed in the United States. In the twentieth and twenty-first centuries it has found its way in both savory and sweet dishes—as an ingredient used in recipes from popular cookbooks.

Banana Cardamom Nut Bread

Weeks after my introduction to cardamom, I put it to use in a birthday bread for my Indian steady. I used a recipe from *Spices of the World Cookbook* by McCormick. The classic nut bread recipe included ground cardamom. Inspired by the twentieth-century tried-and-tested formula, I changed it up with my favorite ingredients (like butter and yogurt) and more spices for the twenty-first-century palate.

2 large eggs, organic
¼ to ½ cup brown sugar
½ cup European-style butter (save a small amount to
*   butter loaf dish)*
2 ripe, large bananas, mashed
1 teaspoon vanilla extract
1½ cups self-rising flour
½ cup Greek yogurt
¼ cup low-fat, organic milk
1 teaspoon cinnamon (McCormick)
½ teaspoon cardamom (McCormick)
½ teaspoon allspice (McCormick)
½ cup chopped walnuts
Confectioners sugar or raw sugar (optional)
Thyme sprigs (for garnish)
Fresh fruit slices (your choice of seasonal fruit)

Preheat the oven to 350 degrees F. In a bowl, combine eggs, sugar, and butter. Blend in the mashed bananas and vanilla. Add flour to the banana mixture. Mix and stir in yogurt, milk, spices, and walnuts. Pour batter into a buttered 9-inch by 6-inch loaf dish. Bake for about 1 hour or until firm to touch. If the top browns too fast, cover with foil after 30 minutes in the oven. Cool for at least 30 minutes. Sprinkle with sugar and thyme. You can serve warm or chilled. Garnish with seasonal fruit slices. I used bananas for late autumn. A pat of butter or raw honey can be a nice touch.

Makes 8 to 10 servings.

CARDAMOM PLANT POWER: SURPRISE STUFF

There are two varieties of cardamom. One is the pods, which come from an Asian shrub that has long pointy leaves and flowers containing the green and white pods with cardamom seeds. Black cardamom, the second type, is a stronger spice (which is in my kitchen cupboard). It has a smoky-peppery-type aroma for super spicy recipes, like chili or hot stews. But you can grind the milder seeds and green seed pods. (I have these pods, which look like pumpkin seeds. But I haven't used them as of yet.)

Like bay leaves, 1,8-cinole plays a role in this spice. The smell of cardamom is from alpha-terpinyl acetate. Interestingly, the Indian variety of cardamom gives us two types—Malabar and Mysore. The latter one boasts more of the potent phytochemical limonene, which has antioxidants that aid in purifying chemicals. Phytonutrient-rich cardamom is good for you, but it's also healthful because of its nutrients.

According to the USDA Nutrient Database, one tablespoon of ground cardamom contains a wide variety of nutrients. It is low cal, with a mere 18 calories, 1.5 grams of dietary fiber, 4 grams of fat, and .6 grams of protein. What's of special interest is that this spice contains a whopping four-fifths of your daily requirement of manganese.

GROUNDBREAKING DISCOVERIES

So, that little compound 1,8 cineole comes to the rescue to fight big respiratory problems. No, it's not heart disease or cancer, but if you have a difficult time breathing, you may be interested in how this chemical in cardamom works for your lungs.

It's a godsend if you have a hacking cough or bronchitis. Research shows the compound acts as an expectorant, which can lessen phlegm allowing you to be less congested. Bronchitis can turn into a pneumonia, which is no laughing matter. A friend of mine had walking pneumonia. She drank a homemade tea, draining the pod seeds; it helped her breathe easier. But antibiotics were prescribed as a precaution, so she recovered sooner.

Bountiful Benefits: Other things cardamom can do is help tummy trouble. It was noted for its help back in ancient times to relieve digestive troubles, according to the Herb Society of America. The strong spice is also believed to stimulate bile flow, which is good for the liver. Dr. Ann Louise Gittleman, a fan of cardamom, agrees this spice can "detoxify and flush out toxins in the liver." Credit may be due to its aromatic compounds, she says, which is helpful during the change of seasons, such as winter to spring. It's the perfect time to "detox pathways," she adds. Not to forget cardamom may also help fat metabolism and help you burn calories. This spice is also praised for its ability to limit mucus. If it works for you it may help guard against pesky sinus congestion and respiratory woes.

Safety Sound Bite: If you have gallstones, pass on this spice.

Shake It Up Now! Cardamom is also used present-day in both cooking and baking. I've added it to spicy cake recipes to provide more flavor. It can be used in a tea drink, like my friend used for medicinal purposes, or Turkish coffee. Mountain Rose Herbs notes they have a wide variety of customers who order this spice and will brew and distill beverages with the full-flavor and strong spice of cardamom.

Not only is this spice used in beverages, but it's found in savory dishes and sweet desserts. It's infused in chocolate truffles and bars! Cardamom oil from the plant is used to flavor pharmaceuticals, and as a fragrance in detergents and body care products like soaps and perfume. There are a variety of makers, one is James Heeley's Esprit du Tigre with notes of cloves and cardamom. It's available in pods, seeds, and ground form available online and in supermarkets.

Libido-Enriching

Cardamom Spicy Pudding

❖ ❖ ❖

Pudding and I go back to childhood when it was baked in the oven. It is one of the desserts I made because it's failproof. Since my growing-up years, during tight times, it's been my signature dish. I adore it—all versions with white or brown rice and a variety of dairy, fruits, and nuts. Pudding is a comfort food—and flavored with cardamom it's even more comforting. This is my recipe, a version spawned by the first romance in my life and inspired by Indian ingredients, including cardamom and saffron. It's a spicy treat to love during colder seasons, and delicious from the first bite, like a first kiss.

1¼ cups brown rice, natural whole grain, cooked (or traditional white rice)
2½ cups organic half-and-half
2 large brown eggs, beaten
¼ cup sugar, pure cane, granulated white
1 teaspoon vanilla extract
½ teaspoon cardamom (McCormick)
1 dash of saffron (The Spice House)
1 teaspoon cinnamon
½ teaspoon nutmeg

TOPPING

½ cup golden raisins
½ cup dried dates
½ cup almonds, chopped
Whipped cream
A dash of nutmeg

Preheat the oven to 325 degrees F. Mix cooked rice and half-and-half in a bowl. Add eggs and sugar. Stir well. Add vanilla and spices. Fold in dried fruit and almonds. Pour into 4 ramekins. Place in an 8-inch by 8-inch dish filled with water. Bake pudding for about 1 hour or until firm. Cool and top with dollop of whipped cream and the dash of nutmeg. Refrigerate. I suggest warming up when you indulge.

Makes 4 to 6 servings.

It wouldn't surprise me if you discover cardamom is one of your favorite spices to put to work in and out of the kitchen. The next exotic spice that'll put heat in your life is not from the Mediterranean countries either. But it is used in European recipes—and its chemical compounds do have amazing healing powers, too.

HEALING HIGHLIGHTS FROM NATURE'S GARDEN-FEST

✓ Cardamom's original roots are derived from India and perhaps Mexican regions. Ancient history shows both Greeks and Egyptians used it for personal hygiene.

✓ ...And today people continue to use it to freshen their breath, guard against respiratory ailments, from coughs to congestion, and worse.

✓ One of its chemical compounds is cineole, which is key to help keep your lungs healthy. It's a great spice if you're blindsided by secondhand smoke or polluted air (from smog to wildfires).

✓ Cardamom, like allspice, has many uses in cooking and baking because of its burst of flavor and can be used in both savory and sweet Mediterranean or Indian dishes.

✓ The seed pods (which you should grind before using to get the most flavor and health benefits) can enhance fresh fruit dishes, rice casseroles, egg custard, or bread pudding.

✓ You can find cardamom in good-for-you superfoods like specialty coffee and tea—and even dark chocolate sprinkled with sea salt.

8

Cayenne

(Solanaceae)

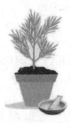

We need the tonic of wildness.
—HENRY DAVID THOREAU

In the seventies, cayenne peppers were part of my spice regime to get lean like fashion models, actors, and fitness gurus. After graduating from high school, I fell into a "flower child" unconventional lifestyle. One autumn afternoon clad in a bell bottom jeans, a cropped sweater, and beads in my braids, I rode my ten-speed bicycle to a Mexican restaurant in Los Gatos. My mission: take-out tortilla chips and hot salsa. It was spiked with fresh cayenne peppers.

Sitting on a bench outdoors, gazing at the Los Gatos foothills, I munched on chips dipped into the spicy sauce. I anticipated visiting my gran in Tucson, Arizona, a region where southwest cuisine included hot cayenne peppers. After savoring the low-cal snack, I gained energy and self-confidence because I didn't overindulge in fattening food. I rode my bike to the park and socialized with friends. We shared our diet secrets. I insisted it was metabolism-boosting salsa that was my new hot secret to staying lean and feeling energized.

THE FAMILY TREE OF CAYENNE

Cayenne's origins are linked to French Guiana, which is in South America. Cayenne did make its way throughout the world, century by century. Credit is doled out to the sea pioneers who brought it back to the old world in the expedition era. A variety of historians claim the first one to allegedly discover cayenne pepper is Christopher Columbus while he was traveling in the Caribbean.

You don't have to look far to discover cayenne was used as a medicinal herb back in the late 1500s and 1600s. And it did make its way to the Mediterranean region. In Europe, it was prescribed to treat skin infections and sore throats. By the nineteenth century, the healing powers of cayenne were used to guard against aches and pains, respiratory conditions, and even mental ailments like depression. Also, cayenne pepper heats up Mediterranean recipes such as sauces and seafood dishes.

In the twentieth century, medical doctors recognized the health benefits of cayenne. In fact, the spicy herb was documented in the *American Illustrated Medical Dictionary*, the *Merck Manual*, and *Materia Medica*. Cayenne was given merit by conventional people in the medical field for its healing powers and it was even available in medicinal products at pharmacies.

CAYENNE PLANT POWER: SURPRISE STUFF

No doubt, it's the capsaicin compound that gets the glory in cayenne for its functional healing powers. Past research in labs have shown this ingredient has antibacterial, anti-carcinogenic, pain-relieving, and anti-diabetic properties. Cayenne contains plenty of flavonoids, like carotenes, lutein, zeaxanthin, and cryptoxanthin. It is capsaicin, though, that gives cayenne its umpteen pain-relieving benefits.

According to the USDA Nutrient Database, cayenne contains plenty of nutrients that will make you happy, too. One teaspoon of cayenne

pepper contains only 16 calories. It has almost half of your needed recommended daily amount of vitamin A. It includes antioxidant vitamins C and E, vitamin K, vitamin B6, manganese, potassium, omega-3
fatty acids, and trace amounts of other essential minerals, like protein
and calcium.

CAYENNE

Nutrition facts for a serving size containing 100 grams (3½ ounces)

Nutrient Value		Percentage of RDA
Calories	337	17
Carbohydrates	50.02 g	38
Protein	12.01 g	21
Cholesterol	0 mg	0
Dietary fiber	27.2 g	71
Folates	106 mcg	26
Vitamins		
Niacin	8.701 mg	54
Pyridoxine	2.450 mg	39
Riboflavin	0.919 mg	71
Thiamin	0.328 mg	27
Vitamin A	41,610 IU	138
Vitamin C	76.4 mg	127
Vitamin E	29.83 mg	199

Vitamin K	80.3 mg	67
Sodium	30 mg	2
Potassium	2014 mg	43
Minerals		
Calcium	148 mg	15
Copper	0.373 mg	41
Iron	7.80 mg	97.5
Magnesium	152 mg	38
Manganese	2.00 mg	87
Phosphorus	293 mg	42
Zinc	2.48 mg	22.5

(Source: USDA Nutrient Database)

Cayenne Pepper: Easy Does It. It's Got Heat!

Welcome to a hot spice that people love but must use with caution when savoring this spicy stuff! Meet Abby Olson, registered dietitian of White Bear Lake, Minnesota, who knows too well about using spices the right and wrong way. Here, take a look at her unforgettable lesson with cayenne. "One of my favorite spices to cook with is cayenne. Cayenne is a pepper from the capsicum family of vegetables, and I love using cayenne. It contains capsaicin, which is the part of the pepper that gives them it's spicy kick," points out Olson, R.D., "and is also the active component that is known for its health benefits.

"I was introduced to cayenne when I started living on my own and took the time to experiment with cooking. I recall the first time I used cayenne in a soup. I realized after tasting the soup that I had gone a little overboard and used a bit too much, and quickly learned my lesson that more is not always better!"

Adds Olson: "I like to keep the dried powder version of cayenne handy so I can reach for a small pinch to add to my dishes. When using a fresh version of a pepper, it is important to wear gloves when cutting and cleaning it, including removing any seeds. Wash your hands before touching your face so you won't burn your skin. Remember a little goes a long way."

These days, Olson, a cayenne proponent, has learned to appreciate the healing powers that herbs and spices can provide. "I love that we are able to utilize these gems from the earth," she adds, "in order to enhance and support health while providing flavor to what we eat and drink."

GROUNDBREAKING DISCOVERIES

Cayenne provides a wealth of healing powers to stave off diseases, including heart disease. Research shows this versatile spice may help to lower blood pressure, keeping your numbers at a healthy level. How? How can a simple spice help to keep your blood pressure normal? Scientists believe cayenne pepper may lower blood pressure thanks to the compound capsaicin. It may help dilate blood vessels and increase blood circulation. More research is needed but for now it seems worth a try. One more thing. Homemade salsa (lose the salt; store-bought varieties can contain a lot) with cayenne pepper is low calorie and low sodium, two other pluses to keep your blood pressure numbers in check.

Scientists also discovered capsaicin pills (the compound in cayenne) may do more for heart health. The chemical compound can boost high-density lipoprotein HDL, the "good" cholesterol, and lower triglyceride numbers (the fat in your body that can cause heart attacks and strokes). When used regularly but in moderation with a healthy diet and exercise it may help lower triglycerides and LDL, "bad" cholesterol, levels. So this is one more piece of the puzzle why cayenne may be heart-healthy.

Bountiful Benefits: I can attest cayenne pepper also works wonders providing ASAP relief for sinus congestion and pressure around the face. I learned this fact from a medical doctor at U.C.L.A., when I was writing about foods that can help fight winter colds and flu. Cayenne also gets kudos for its ability to lessen joint and muscle pain, which can pay you a visit if you catch a virus.

I discovered that cayenne pepper in salsa is a good sinus-clearing aid when traveling. At Salt Lake City, Utah, airport when I am laid-over waiting for a flight inbound or outbound, it's a must-have congestion cure like when the salsa healed my sinus headache. Speaking of pain, I penned a self-help article on 10 natural pain relievers. Cayenne was in the mix. Why? Credit is given to the compound capsaicin, which depletes substance P, a brain chemical that creates inflammation and sends "ouch, I'm feeling pain" messages to the brain. No surprise, capsaicin is an ingredient in anti-pain topical creams.

Olson praises cayenne, along with other nutrition experts, for the anti-inflammatory benefits as it contains antioxidants that fight free radicals, which can do damage to the body cells and cause diseases. She also knows as I do about its pain-reducing perks when used topically, how it can be used as an immune booster, and its benefit as an aid in digestion because it stimulates gastric juices and digestive enzymes, so our bodies digest properly.

Shake It Up Now! Cayenne is very versatile and readily available. It can be used in powder form for convenience to be stored in your spice cabinet. Fresh cayenne peppers in the fridge are wonderful, especially for cooking. Cayenne is also an ingredient in dark chocolate truffles and bars. I've been known to indulge in a Lake Champlain Chocolates Spicy Aztec Bar every so often. It is 57 percent cacao and contains both bold cayenne pepper and cinnamon. The cayenne adds gusto to the semi-sweet chocolate.

Cayenne pepper is also available in topical pain-relieving medicinal creams and even bandages. It can be used in tea and is available in capsules as a supplement.

Safety Sound Bite: Consuming cayenne can trigger heartburn. This isn't a surprise, since it ranks high on the hot foods Scoville Rating Scale: 30,000 to 190,000 Scoville Heat Units.

Anti-Inflammatory

Cayenne Spicy Salsa and Greek Baked Chips

Salsa is a favorite food of mine. After a book signing with a small turnout of people in the San Francisco Bay Area, I was feeling down. At a Mexican food restaurant, I was seated and served a basket of warm tortilla chips and smooth salsa. The intense flavor and heat took my mind off the day that my welcome home celebration tanked. I often make homemade chunky salsa, but one spring day in my cabin at Lake Tahoe, I go nostalgic for the smooth stuff. This delicious and cayenne hot salsa is a tribute to the dive that will always have a place in my heart wherever I am.

2 cups tomatoes, fresh, diced (I used Roma variety)
¼ cup onion, yellow or red, chopped
¼ cup jalapeno pepper, seeded, diced
2 teaspoons fresh garlic clove, minced
2 teaspoons fresh cilantro, chopped
½ teaspoon herbes de Provence
½ teaspoon cayenne pepper
A dash of ground pepper and sea salt to taste
2 teaspoons fresh lemon juice

In a blender or a food processor combine tomatoes, onion, jalapeno pepper, garlic, herbs, spices, and lemon juice. Blend until smooth. Put into plastic container, cover. Chill in fridge for at least one hour.

GREEK BAKED CHIPS

Six whole grain pita pockets
Olive oil or canola oil (for drizzling)
1 teaspoon Italian seasoning
Ground lemon pepper to taste (Mountain Rose Herbs)

Preheat the oven to 350 degrees F. Cut pita pocket circles in half. Slice into triangles. Place triangles on a nonstick baking sheet. Drizzle with oil. Sprinkle with Italian seasoning and pepper. Bake several minutes until golden. Turn once. Remove when golden brown and crispy. Serve hot with salsa.

Serves 4.

It's time to put the cayenne spice wonder back on the spice rack and bring on a versatile herb to love. Welcome to chives, a lovely mild herb. Let me show you the varied reasons why this under-rated herb made my top 22 list—and it just may make the cut for you, too. It's time to meet the little green herbal underdog.

HEALING HIGHLIGHTS FROM NATURE'S GARDEN-FEST

✓ First and foremost, this hot herb is heart-healthy. Don't forget it can help dilate blood vessels and boost circulation, which is actually good for your ticker at any age.

✓ Another focal point of this herb is its capsaicin, which is helpful if you're watching your cholesterol and/or want to keep those numbers under control.

✓ If you fall victim to seasonal allergies and/or sinus problems, rest assured cayenne is your friend. It can zap congestion, clear the airways. Add this herb to your favorite salads, sauces, dips, and vegetables—and breathe easy!

✓ The chemical compound capsaicin is the WORD for you if you face aches and pains and want relief, naturally. If you hurt, RUN don't walk to the drugstore and grab an over-the-counter anti-inflammatory cream with c-a-p-s-a-i-c-i-n. Got it?

✓ If you're wanting to rev up that snail-like metabolism due to hormones or age, cayenne is for you. (Turn to the chapter "Season Up, Slim Down" and you'll find out how it works to help your body to burn calories FAST!)

Chives

(Liliaceae)

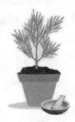

Oh, better no doubt is a dinner of herbs
When season'd with love, which no rancour disturbs
And sweetene'd by all that is sweetest in life
Than turbot, bisque, ortolans, eaten in strife!
—EDWARD BULWER-LYTTON, "Lucile" (1860)

Sweet chives found their way into my life during my first round at college on a study date with a fellow student. We both were on a struggling, starving student budget. Salad bars were a huge phenomenon back in the seventies (and were still popular before the pandemic). As a vegetarian (on rare occasion I do eat fish), adding herby flavor to vegetables was still new to me. My food-savvy friend took charge of my plate. On a large russet baked potato, he added green chives, a dash of cayenne, and ground pepper.

"Wow!" I exclaimed when taking a bite bursting with flavor. My date smiled. He quoted the well-known author Louisa May Alcott: "Money is the root of evil, and yet it is such a useful root that we cannot get on without it any more than we can without potatoes." The words resonated with me because of my rolling pennies and eating potatoes and salads days. And that was the night I remember chives, a mild onion-like flavor entered my life.

The green herb revisited me throughout the decades, like a long-lost love—a prodigal perfect herb to enhance a simple dish. Fresh chives (homegrown or in the organic produce store aisle) are my favorite herb sprinkled on potato skins and baby spinach salads. Dried chives in a glass jar suffice when sprinkled on a solo baked potato with crucifers and a dollop of European-style butter. I learned that a chive-less tater is like a slice of hot apple pie without a scoop of vanilla ice cream.

THE FAMILY TREE OF CHIVES

Did you know chives are relatives to garlic, onions, and shallots? It makes sense to me since I adore all three for many reasons. My food relationship with the trio goes back decades in my life, and they have a long history.

Chives go back to 3000 B.C., according to the Herb Society of America, who add they have roots in Europe, Central Asia, and North America. Chives were used by the Romans for some health ailments, such as sore throats and sunburn, but they didn't receive the same love that garlic did. Marco Polo, claims the HSA, is believed to have brought the healing herb to Europe from China in the late 1400s.

Chives began to get their recognition in the 1800s, when they were used in European cooking. Countries like France, Poland, and Sweden included the little green onion-flavored herb in soups and sandwiches.

CHIVES PLANT POWER: SURPRISE STUFF

So, chives win in the phenolic compound department over its nutrient power. Its phytonutrients are workhorses, and scientists suggest they contain anti-inflammatory, antibiotic, and anti-viral properties. It's the bioflavonoids that may contain cancer-fighting properties.

While the chemical compounds in chives are noteworthy—chives also contain disease-fighting antioxidant vitamins A, C, and E. Not to forget chives contain some bone-building calcium, iron, and zinc. If paired with nutritious foods, such as potassium-rich potatoes, these mild onion-flavored green herbs enhance a dish and titillate your taste buds.

GROUNDBREAKING DISCOVERIES

First and foremost, those chives rich in bioflavonoids include organosulfide, which scientific lab studies suggest may guard against cancers, including colorectal, prostate, and stomach. More research is needed before we can say for sure.

And if you pair chives with nutrient-dense vegetables, like I did in the student union at the salad bar, it's a good thing. Food researchers do know nutritious, colorful fruits and vegetables are on the cutting edge of being prescribed by our medical doctors. In fact, health practitioners and nutritionists do advise people to eat more produce.

Bountiful Benefits: Since chives contain many chemical compounds, it can heal many health ailments. Chives may help with arthritis or fibromyalgia aches and pains, thanks to its anti-inflammatory properties. Also, its antifungal benefits may be helpful to stave off a common cold or even a pesky bout of flatulence. Not to be underestimated its bioflavonoids may help to keep those blood pressure numbers at a healthy reading, naturally.

Incorporating fresh or dried chives into healthful fare, such as baked potatoes and vegetable casseroles, will help you to get the phytonutrients in vegetables. Both the American Cancer Society and American Heart Association recommend you consume fruit and vegetables daily.

Shake It Up Now! Chives are found readily available in supermarket foods, including cream cheese, chips, crackers, and breads. If I am on the road and stop at a drive-thru, a baked potato with chives at the popular Wendy's is a must-have. I've use dried chives for convenience in baking scones and cornbread. However, fresh chives sprinkled on scrambled eggs or soups are even tastier. Chive edible flowers can be grown in your garden or available at grocery stores. You can separate the flowers into florets and add them to fresh salads, eggs, and soups. Fresh chives (homegrown or found in the organic produce grocery store aisle) are my favorite herb sprinkled on potato skins. Dried chives (on a cold winter's night) when sprinkled onto a shepherd's pie—a poor man's feast—is a comforting complete meal.

Pound-Paring

Beef Tenderloin with Chives and Parsley (Topped with Red Wine Demi Sauce)

Herbs and spices play a big role at health resorts. Guests often want to lose weight. It's nutritious foods, portion control, and flavor that come to the rescue. I learned years ago, while interviewing posh spas from California to New York, that lean protein and seasonings are a chef's wonder tool. Meat in moderation is part of the Mediterranean diet. What's more, carnivores (yes, I understand not everyone can give up beef) will love a savory dish seasoned with fresh herbs. This recipe is created by a well-known chef who indeed puts Mediterranean cuisine and nature's chives and parsley to work.

MARINATED BEEF TENDERLOIN

1 tablespoon grapeseed oil
2 tablespoons chopped fresh parsley
2 tablespoons chopped fresh chives
Kosher or sea salt and freshly ground pepper
4 beef tenderloin fillets (4 ounces each), cut 3-inches
*   thick*

In a small bowl, combine the oil, parsley, and chives. Salt and pepper the beef fillets. Rub the marinade over the beef and marinate for 2 hours in the refrigerator.

RED WINE DEMI SAUCE

2 tablespoons grapeseed oil
1 onion, sliced
2 ribs celery, peeled and sliced
2 carrots, trimmed, peeled, and sliced
2 tablespoons tomato paste
2 cups dry red wine
4 cups beef or veal stock
Sea salt

In a large saucepan over medium heat, add the oil, onions, celery, and carrots. Sauté for about 10 minutes, stirring often, until the vegetables are caramelized and dark in color. Add the tomato paste and cook until it turns a brick red color. And the red wine, bring to a boil, and then reduce the heat to a simmer. When reduced in volume by half, add the beef or veal stock and continue to cook at a simmer until a syrup-like consistency is achieved. Strain the vegetables from the sauce and season with salt to taste. Set aside and keep warm.

Tenderloin Preparation

Marinated Beef Tenderloins
2 teaspoons grapeseed oil

Preheat the oven to 350 degrees F. Remove the tenderloins from the refrigerator, take out of the marinade and pat dry with paper towels. Let sit for about 30 minutes so they will come to room temperature. In a large oven-safe sauté pan over medium-high heat, add the grapeseed oil. Sear the first side of the tenderloins for about a minute, or until they're golden brown color. Flip the fillets over and sear the other sides. Transfer to the oven and cook for about 5 minutes for a medium finish. Remove from the oven and let rest for 5 minutes. To serve, place one tenderloin on each plate with Mashed Sweet Potatoes with Paprika. (See the chapter "Paprika.") Top with the Red Wine Demi Sauce. Add greens of your choice.

Serves 4.

(Courtesy: Chef Curtis Cooke, Cal-a-Vie Havens, Terri and John, *Beautiful Living: Cooking the Cal-A-Vie Health Spa Way*)

Now that you've got the goods on chives, we're moving along to another popular herb—cilantro. It's a superstar when cooking it up in dishes because it's healthful and has a distinct flavor. Got your interest? Come on, let me show you my findings!

Healing Highlights From Nature's Garden-Fest

✓ Be aware that chives do more than flavor up a baked potato. Why? They have a combo of phytonutrients that can guard you against some diseases . . .

✓ Enter heart health. Yes, chives, like onions, are heart-healthy, especially if you use them more than less to add aroma and taste to salads, soups, vegetables, and fish to meat.

✓ It's the antioxidants in this herb that guard your body against in-flammation and environmental culprits.

✓ Check out foods and recipes that include chives—fresh or dried—and discover how versatile this flavorful herb can be.

✓ You can use dried chives in baking and fresh chives are preferred to top on cooked food.

Cilantro

(Umbelliferae)

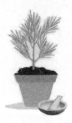

*Some writers say the leaves [cilantro] are used for
seasoning, but this statement seems odd, as all the green
parts of the plant exhale a very strong odor and of the
wood-bug, whence the Greek name of the plant.*
—VILMOUN-ANDRIA X, *The Vegetable Garden* (1885)

Cilantro is another superherb, known for its super versatility used in a
variety of regions and cuisines. A man in my life, with a Lady
Macbeth–type domineering mother in tow, introduced me to bittersweet cilantro. One summer day, in our rental house, the entertaining
but manipulative mom made bruschetta topped with tomato and
cilantro. The ingredients included artisan French bread topped with
chopped onion, garlic, Roma tomatoes, cheeses, and it was decorated
with cilantro.

I mumbled, "This green stuff tastes like soap." She darted, "Your
palate is childlike." Her son laughed at her observation as I picked off

the herb, one by one, like a vegetarian does with salami on a pizza. She took a bite out of the appetizer and added, "You don't own a pot to cook in." As a self-professed, sophisticated foodie, she knew how to cook gourmet dishes using herbs for aroma and flavor, reminding me of a competitive celebrity chef on TV. Once she even raved about my cayenne-zested shrimp risotto. On the cilantro day I felt like my culinary knowledge plummeted below the fry guy at the local food drive-thru. It was the beginning of the end for a wilting relationship; but I moved on to learning to enhance herbs—like fresh cilantro.

After my initiation to cilantro, my nutrition class professor taught me about the health benefits of the ancient herb I refused to eat. What did I know? I was just a naïve student living on pasta and bland marinara sauce in a jar. So, the Shakespearean-type strong-willed woman was right. I was wrong. The silver lining was I ended up getting a cookware set (with pots) so I, too, could learn to prepare dishes with cilantro—and like it. As time passed, I appreciated the citrusy aroma of cilantro, but it's an acquired taste.

THE FAMILY TREE OF CILANTRO

History shows that cilantro goes back to 5000 B.C. The plant was grown in ancient Egypt and used by both Greeks and Romans. It was used as a medicinal herb and used in tombs. Cilantro's origin is the eastern Mediterranean regions, according to the Herb Society of America. In the Medieval era, adds the society, the seeds and leaves had culinary benefits.

Interestingly, the HSA and herbalists say, "cilantro and coriander are the same plant." The leaves and stems of cilantro are used in cooking. The seeds, which are referred to as coriander, may be used whole, crushed, or ground. Both the seeds and leaves, adds HSA, have been used since ancient times.

Historical sources believe in the mid-1700s liquor was made from coriander seeds.

It is said that this leafy herb was one of the first plants grown by colonists. Like my past love-hate relationship with the herb, it can have a citrusy aroma to some, while others claim it smells like soap. It is an acquired taste, but the truth is I adore it and for many reasons it deserves kudos in my book.

CILANTRO PLANT POWER: SURPRISE STUFF

Like other leafy garden herbs, this one does boast some good-for-you nutrients. Cilantro provides phytonutrients, such as flavonoids, which include epigenin, kaempferol, rhamnetin, and quercetin. Quercetin, for one, gives cilantro its healing powers because of its antioxidant abilities, which may guard you against cancer and heart disease. Also, the compound Borneol has the ability to zap germs and viruses—a plus especially during cold and flu season or if you're traveling and exposed to a lot of microbes sitting on surfaces in aircraft, restaurants, and public restrooms.

Also, the ancient herb is a dieter's best friend since it's super low-cal, has no dietary fat, no sodium, and no cholesterol. Fresh cilantro leaves do contain vitamin K, which plays a role in helping to keep your bones strong. One-fourth cup cilantro contains approximately 14 percent of a woman's daily recommended amount; 10 percent for a man. Evidently, dried cilantro doesn't provide you with as much vitamin K, so when possible use fresh cilantro in your recipes.

GROUNDBREAKING DISCOVERIES

Due to the antioxidant quercetin in cilantro, past scientific research hints that cilantro may help guard against cancer and heart disease. This chemical compound is known to help bolster the immune and cardiovascular systems, so it strengthens the body. It's the antioxidants in cilantro, just like in other herbs, that work to protect your body against free radicals.

Other research hints that polyphenols and heart-healthy factors, like no saturated fat in cilantro, may help heart health. Also, some scientific findings suggest cilantro in your diet may lower LDL or "bad" cholesterol, and even boost HDL or "good" cholesterol. More research is needed for hard-hitting proof. For now, using a heart-healthy Mediterranean diet and combining it with healthy foods and the herb cilantro can do a body good—especially your heart.

Bountiful Benefits: Cilantro contains antimicrobial properties, so it can help detoxify the body from tainted foods. This herb also may lessen anxiety (I wish I knew that when served the bruschetta by my ex's mom). Other health perks of cilantro include keeping blood sugar levels steady, which can stave off type 2 diabetes, and including this herb in your diet and lifestyle may heal skin inflammation.

Shake It Up Now! This herb is used in cooking different cuisines, from Mediterranean to Mexican. It is available fresh at the supermarket. I have purchased it fresh in organic form packaged, and dried to add to my collection of herbs. You can get your fix of superfood cilantro in a variety of ways, including lime cilantro bath bombs, essential oil, and even capsule supplements available online.

Anti-Inflammatory

Cilantro Cheesy Pull-Apart Bread

❖ ❖ ❖

This recipe is inspired by the bruschetta I was served and the cilantro I tossed due to ignorance. I was not enjoying the adventure of trying new herbs! Years later, when shopping at the local grocery store, I picked up a round loaf of artisan bread. It was wintertime when the body craves hot, comfort food such as bread and cheese. I put together this easy recipe and wow! I was pleasantly surprised at the amazing flavors of the herbs and spices. I dedicate this cilantro treat to the woman who taught me to open my mind and mouth to new and interesting foods.

½ cup or stick of European-style butter, melted
¼ cup parsley, fresh
¼ cup cilantro, fresh
1 teaspoon garlic clove, minced
Ground black pepper to taste
¼ cup each cheddar, mozzarella, Parmesan cheese
    shavings, chopped
1 small 12-inch by 12-inch round artisan sourdough
    bread

Preheat the oven to 350 degrees F. In a bowl, melt butter in microwave. Add parsley, cilantro, garlic, and pepper. Slice the top of the bread in horizontal and vertical lines to create crevices. Drizzle the butter herb mixture on top and allow it to drip into the cut holes. Stuff cheese pieces into the openings. Place bread onto foil and cover. Put on a baking sheet. Bake 15 minutes until cheese is melted. Remove top foil. Turn up heat to 400 degrees F and bake about 10 more minutes until cheese bubbles and top of bread is golden. Remove from oven. Serve immediately.

Serves 6 to 8.

It's time to take cilantro off the table and bring in cloves. You'll discover the wonders of this intriguing spice that is healthful and can flavor up your food.

HEALING HIGHLIGHTS FROM NATURE'S GARDEN-FEST

✓ Do note, while cilantro is often used in Mexican cuisine it is also paired with foods from the Mediterranean diet.
✓ Some herbalists claim cilantro's origin is unknown; other sources including the Herbal Society of America believe the herb is native to the Mediterranean region.
✓ Cilantro are the leaves and coriander the seeds—but they are from the same plant.
✓ Psst! Do think of cilantro as more than a garnish. This herb contains nutrients and chemical compounds that are good for your health.
✓ . . . It contains about 30 percent of your daily requirement for vitamin K—a forgotten gem that is needed for good blood health and more.
✓ Cilantro is one of those herbs that you'll either love or take a while to appreciate its distinct flavor.

Cloves

(Myrtaceae)

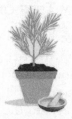

Now no joy but lacks salt. That is not dashed with
pain And weariness and fault; I crave the stain Of
tears, the aftermark Of almost too much love,
The sweet bitter bark And burning clove.
—ROBERT FROST, *To Earthword, a Poem*

I may have lacked cilantro savoir-faire, but my mother, my mentor, showed me the ropes of how to utilize aromatic cloves, a utilitarian spice, at a young age. When I was a kid, I anticipated my mom's full-course dinners created for special occasions, including Easter Sunday. One year, I helped make a picture-perfect cranberry glazed ham with cloves, a spice all lined up like the tips of crayons in a box.

My mom used the Ocean Spray holiday ham recipe, which included a can of jellied cranberry sauce and brown sugar. Once the ham was almost baked, I watched my mother use a knife to create a crosshatch design on top of the meat. My job? Like a carpenter, I imagined, I tacked brown peppery-smelling cloves (resembling tiny brown nails, which are derived from the Latin word *clavus*) onto pineapple rings and whole cherries. Once done, the tic-tac-toe row display was stunning. It was a flawless piece of art, both decorative and fun. I thought, "The ham looks like an armadillo with its natural armor coat." This was my first introduction to the aromatic and peppery hot clove, which I tasted and liked, sort of. As an adult, I haven't changed my mind.

THE FAMILY TREE OF CLOVES

The roots of cloves, a spice likely in your kitchen cabinet, come from the flower bud of the myrtle tree family, grown in Indonesia. Cloves are the bud of the flower, which keeps its distinct peppery aroma and flavor intact. Historians will tell you the strong scent of this spice is what lured explorers to the Spice Islands, islands sandwiched by the Indian and Pacific Oceans.

Medicinal uses of cloves go way back to the Middle Ages. It was one of the ingredients used in the Four Thieves antiseptic formula, which is believed to have had anti-viral and antibacterial protection against the deadly black plague. History also points to Chinese medicine putting cloves, a medicinal aid, to work topically over the stomach. The theory was that the spice can help to aid digestion.

CLOVES PLANT POWER: SURPRISE STUFF

Little cloves pack a powerful punch with their chemical compounds. Remember eugenol, the potent compound found in bay leaf? It is one of the primary heart-healthy compounds in cloves. Other noteworthy chemical compounds include methlamylketone and methysalicylate.[1]

Yes, cloves contain nutrients, too. One teaspoon of cloves holds approximately 15 milligrams of calcium, the mineral we need for strong teeth and bones. It also contains about 25 milligrams of potassium, another mineral found in fruit that balances the sodium in our bodies, good for heart health. Cloves are a good source of dietary fiber, which keeps type 2 diabetes at bay and helps keep us regular. Most shocking, 1 teaspoon of cloves contains a whopping 55 percent of the daily recommended value of manganese, the key nutrient that we need to keep our bones strong.

GROUNDBREAKING DISCOVERIES

Since cloves rank high for their ORAC value (remember I showed their antioxidant status in the first chapter), it's no surprise this spice is antimicrobial, antifungal, and anti-viral. These benefits certainly can help guard you against contagious diseases by bolstering your immune system and cardiovascular system. Here's proof:

Eugenol in clove oil (often the plant oil or extract used in scientific studies because it's more potent) has been reported in the *British Journal of Pharmacology* that it may dilate arteries in the body while simultaneously lowering systemic blood pressure (includes systolic pressure and diastolic pressure). This, in turn, means cloves may help you get a healthier blood pressure reading. As always, more research is needed before any definitive conclusion is made. For now, eating one or two small cloves per day could be helpful.[2]

Bountiful Benefits: Cloves are multipurpose like other spices. This distinct smelling spice is anti-viral so it can help guard against a flu bug. These cuties are also useful to relieve congestion and even work as an air freshener. And who can forget the seventies' film *Marathon Man* when oil of cloves was the must-have antidote for Dustin Hoffman's agonizing toothache. Research shows that cloves are also good for fighting bacteria, including E. coli and staph.

Shake It Up Now! Cloves can also be baked with poultry and meat and also fruits and vegetables. It can be used in ground and whole form, or the essential oil like I have. The clove of essential oil vial sits in my bathroom cabinet just in case a gum or tooth issue happens on a weekend or the end of the world is near. It can also be used in tea for aromatherapy. Autumn spice coffees and teas with artificial and natural flavoring of cloves are delicious. (Refer to the Herbal Healings chapter on how to use cloves for oral ailments.)

Antibacterial

Clove-Honey Glazed Ham

❖ ❖ ❖

Here's another one of my mom's favorite twentieth-century recipes. I gave it a re-do for fun and health's sake. The presentation is pretty and fresh, with a honey spin and no canned pineapple rings or cherries in a jar. Fresh fruit please. This spicy ham is a good meat lover's dish to make, and if lean, it is included in the Mediterranean diet.

1 (8-pound) ham, trimmed of fat
20 whole cloves (The Spice House)
¾ cup raw clover honey
¼ cup brown sugar
¼ cup apricot preserves
¼ cup European-style butter, melted
1 teaspoon thyme
1 teaspoon cinnamon
Pineapple chunks and cherries sliced, fresh

Bake ham according to direction on packaging. About 30 minutes before ham is cooked, remove from oven and get rid of fat from pan. Score ham crisscross with a knife. Place cloves on top. About 20 minutes before the ham is cooked, in a saucepan combine honey, brown sugar, preserves, butter, thyme, and cinnamon. Simmer until melted. Spread half of honey mixture with a pastry brush on top of ham for about 10 minutes, remove the ham from the oven. Spread ham with rest of honey mixture. Top with fresh pineapple and cherries. Bake ham for about 10 more minutes or until golden brown. Do not burn.

Serves 10.

We are now leaving the land of cloves and encountering a medicinal herb called cumin. You may, like me, have enjoyed it in vegetable dishes. But soon you'll find out that cumin, the seed or powder, is so much more than an aromatic plant. Let's move on.

HEALING HIGHLIGHTS FROM NATURE'S GARDEN-FEST

✓ The pungent smell and flavor in little brown cloves are due to their primary chemical component eugenol, found in many other spices.

✓ And eugenol is the compound that gets credit for cloves possibly being heart-healthy, including regulating blood pressure.

✓ In real life both the oil and whole cloves can be applied to numb a toothache or gum irritation.

✓ Cloves are immunity-boosting, which can help guard you against colds, flu, and maybe even cancer.

✓ Both whole cloves and ground powder can be used in cooking and baking—and you will reap health benefits from both forms.

Cumin

(*Umbelliferae*)

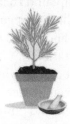

Does he not level its surface And sow dill and scatter
cumin. And Plant wheat in rows, Barley in its place
and rye within its area?
—ISAIAH 28:25, *Thematic Bible*

I didn't have an encounter with cumin until my spicy nomadic adventures in Oregon. At age twenty-two, the kitchen was my refuge. When cooking or baking, ingredients and tools were limited, so creating a culinary delight was a challenge. As a devout vegetarian, I made sad meatless tacos and only used basics: shells, tomatoes, red onion, and lettuce. Not a Portland fish meal to write home about but doable for myself and S.O.

"It's okay," nit-picked my ex-friend I left in Eugene. "You ought to taste my sister's seasoned fish tacos. They're mind-blowing." I rolled my eyes at him. How rude! Because of our bohemian lifestyle I couldn't afford fish or an array of seasonings; and I was clueless anyhow to which herbs and spices could have made a delectable taco. I vowed one day I would learn how to be a gastronome. Once back home in Northern California, a mecca of herbs and spices, I discovered how to spice up foods.

THE FAMILY TREE OF CUMIN

Not unlike other spices, food historians claim spicy cumin has roots in Egypt. There are regular cumin and black cumin seeds, which are smaller and not surprisingly darker in color. The useful spice was also cultivated in other countries, including the Mediterranean.

Cumin was valuable in yesteryear. The spice was surprisingly used to pay taxes, like pepper, and even accepted as contribution to churches. Since it was available to both the Greeks and Romans, it ended up being a cost-effective substitute for pricey pepper. It was used for embalming and was even used to preserve King Tut. But its uses don't end there—there's much more to the lovely spice.

Cumin Love

Speaking of lovely, it's no secret to herbalists that cumin seeds have a history of potential aphrodisiac qualities. Cumin seeds gained popularity for their promise of passion during the Middle Ages. The spice had a reputation of boosting loyalty, and even staving off infidelity. It was rumored that the lovers of fighters were given cumin bread to help them fight against the temptation to be unfaithful when their loves were deployed. What's more, at weddings, guests would keep the little love seeds as a keepsake. Food experts note that an Arabic cumin paste with sweet honey and hot pepper was in demand for increasing ardor.

Cumin Plant Power: Surprise Stuff

Yes, cumin seeds do contain chemical compounds. Some of these are cuminaldehyde, cymene, and terpenoids. It is terpenoids that provide the spicy aroma of cumin seeds. Also, this compound may affect the brain's feel-good chemicals, such as dopamine and serotonin. These are triggered by sunshine, exercise, dark chocolate, and even making love. That means in an instant these little black seeds can put you in a good mood!

I'm not going to tell you cumin is chock-full of essential vitamins and minerals. But it does have some swell nutrients—like iron (a must for vegan and vegetarians, like me). One tablespoon of cumin seeds has a mere 23 calories, 1 gram fat, almost sodium-free, and no sugar. Also, these little seeds boast an entire gram of dietary fiber, and almost one-fourth of your daily value of iron.

Groundbreaking Discoveries

Does cumin have remarkable healing powers? Past research shows cumin supplements can improve blood cholesterol. How? It could be due to the mix of antioxidants. We do know good cholesterol helps lower our risk of developing heart attacks and strokes.

It's not definitive if adding cumin to our diet has the same effect as supplements, though. While the jury is still out, it may be worth it to use a dash of cumin in your diet. Its flavorful taste will entice you to eat fish, a known heart-healthy food with good-for-you omega fatty acids.

Bountiful Benefits: People who like cumin likely know it's a good digestion aid. It may also help detoxify the liver, which is essential, especially if you've overindulged in alcohol or fatty foods. Indian doctors believe cumin has cooling properties that may help lessen heartburn. It is also used for a wide range of allergies.

Shake It Up Now! It is advised to grind whole cumin seeds before serving to get its full flavor. The cumin seeds can also be boiled and steeped in water and served as tea. Cumin is found in spice blends available at the grocery store and Asian specialty shops. It is a culinary spice used for cooking and baking, adding an earthy flavor to food. Cumin black seed oil is also used as an ingredient in anti-aging face creams and essential oil, which can be found online. And note, cumin, like licorice-like anise, can be overpowering so it is recommended to use only a dash in dishes.

Antioxidant-Rich

Tacos with Chicken and Cumin Dressing

When I make dishes, like tacos, I will cook up poultry for carnivore devotees. The extra cost and effort are worth the flavor boost. This Cumin Dressing recipe is my creation paired with a Tacos with Chicken recipe created by my friend Gemma Sciabica, who used down-to-earth European flair, including herbs, spices, Greek yogurt, and olive oil—Mediterranean superfoods.

FOR THE DRESSING

½ cup sour cream
½ cup Greek yogurt, plain
2 teaspoons ground cumin, toasted (in a hot pan for a
    few minutes)
1 teaspoon cayenne pepper
1 teaspoon minced garlic
2 tablespoons fresh lemon juice

In a blender, mix the sour cream, yogurt, cumin, cayenne, garlic, and lemon juice. Blend until smooth. Chill in refrigerator until serving.

FOR THE TACOS WITH CHICKEN

¼ cup Marsala Olive Fruit Oil
1 onion, chopped

1 red bell pepper, sliced thin (or minced)
4 garlic cloves, minced
3 tomatoes
Salt and pepper to taste
¼ teaspoon cumin (or to taste)
½ cup fresh cilantro, chopped
3 to 4 cups chicken, cooked, shredded
8 to 10 taco shells
½ head iceberg lettuce, shredded
2 avocadoes, diced
6 ounces Monterey Jack or Cheddar cheese, shredded
Yogurt or sour cream to taste

In skillet, add oil, onions, peppers, and garlic, cook until crisp tender. Stir in tomatoes, salt, pepper, cumin, and cilantro, cook about 4 to 5 minutes. Add chicken, heat through. Fill taco shells with chicken mixture. Serve lettuce, avocado, cheese, yogurt, or sour cream in separate bowls, add to tacos as desired. (You can skip the yogurt or sour cream and drizzle with Cumin Dressing or use both!)

Serves 8 to 10.

(Courtesy: Gemma Sanita Sciabica, *Cooking with California Olive Oil: Popular Recipes*)

Now that I've tempted you with the pluses of cumin, it's time to introduce another ancient herb called dill. My mom kept it in the pantry to use for cooking purposes. I have it in my kitchen cupboard, too—but it can do so much more. Introducing dill! Drum roll please.

HEALING HIGHLIGHTS FROM NATURE'S GARDEN-FEST

✓ Cumin is a spicy wonder that boasts many perks. It deserves more attention than it gets.

✓ After all, cumin can help you stay heart-healthy. Note: Heart disease does not discriminate. Any age or gender of people can face heart conditions.

✓ This versatile medicinal spice is also good for belly pain, such as IBS and digestion—and it may help you get needed sleep, important for all generations.

✓ Don't forget research suggests cumin may help keep your blood sugar levels steady so you can guard against type 2 diabetes.

✓ Cumin provides a variety of remedies for health ailments, such as boosting happiness because of its ability to trigger feel-good hormones in the body.

✓ Yes, cumin is essential in cooking up adventurous foods—which attracts millennials and boomers for the enhanced flavor and fun—but discover how it also has therapeutic benefits.

Dill

(Umbelliferae)

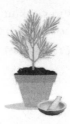

*Woe to you, scribes and Pharisees, hypocrites! For you
tithe mint and dill and cummin, and have neglected the
weightier provision of the law: Justice and mercy and
faithfulness; but these are the things you should have
done without neglecting the others.*
—MATTHEW: 23:23, *New Testament*

Not unlike bay leaf, dill weed brings back fond memories. My first
taste of dill was munching on a homemade cold dill pickle dipped in
spicy mustard. But it was in my mid-twenty-something chapter of life
that I had a summertime dill adventure that still lingers in my mind.
One day while basking in the sun on a raft in the Stanislaus River in
north-central California, I was spotted by a Hemingway-looking man—
a local. He had visited me, time to time, throughout my carefree days
camping on the river.

He was clad in khaki shorts, had a tanned body and face, complete with a bushy white beard. I heard his words, "The wife made you lunch." I with dog in tow rowed to shore. On the sand was a rustic basket. I opened up the lid and was greeted with cold fried chicken paired with a plastic container of herbed potato salad. The green and brown specks teased a hint of deliciousness. I tasted the feathery dill weed, the herb my mom used in making homemade pickles. The man shouted, "Seize the day!" His words echoed as he walked up the stairs to his two-story house with decorative patio umbrellas and a docked boat. He left me, an image of Huckleberry Finn on the water, to eat the food flavored with an array of herbs to be savored. I still have memories of that day on the river when I was living in the present. And yes, I took the time to smell the dill (much like the adage goes for roses), with its fine, delicate leaf, in a salad.

THE FAMILY TREE OF DILL

Herbalists and historians alike agree that dill weed, which is in the plant family of the bay leaf and cumin, was discovered in Egypt five thousand years ago. It has roots of being used as a medicinal herb in the Mediterranean countries since the Middle Ages. It has been noted that Charlemagne or Charles the Great, the King of Italy and the Roman Emperor, used it in flower arrangements. On his food table-space it was available for guests who overindulged because of its digestive aid qualities. Also, a note to myself: Dill was believed to be a symbol of abundance. I wonder if this superstition still holds true.

DILL PLANT POWER: SURPRISE STUFF

The flowers, leaves, and seeds from dill have been used for many purposes centuries ago and present-day. All three forms can be used as a culinary herb in cooking and baking. Dill leaves are more subtle in flavor. Dill weed refers to its leaves while the word "dill" means its seeds.

Like other herbs, sweetish dill has antioxidant value that makes it a powerhouse of goodness. Dill contains many healing compounds; however, its major players are monoterpenes, including limonene, carvone, anethofuran, and flavonoids vicenin and kaempferol.

Dill also contains essential minerals, and certain amino acids that are in both its seeds and leaves. Some of these include vitamin A and C, folate, iron, and manganese. Interestingly, its flavor can contain hints of caraway, lemon, and parsley.

GROUNDBREAKING DISCOVERIES

Can dill work as an antidepressant *and* pain reliever? Maybe. A study published in the *American Journal of Therapeutics* discovered dill extract contains antidepressant and analgesic properties compared to the drugs tramadol and sertraline. And dill doesn't come with the side effects of antidepressants.[1]

With kudos to all of dill's antioxidants, it's no surprise that it is touted by scientists to have anti-cancer, anti-diabetes, and anti-stress benefits. Dill is believed to be helpful in guarding against metabolic syndrome (a combination of high blood pressure, cholesterol, sugar levels, and obesity). More research is needed but because of its disease-fighting properties dill still shows promise as a healthful herb.

Bountiful Benefits: The consensus among herbalists is that dill is a super digestive aid. That means it can soothe an upset stomach and help relieve the discomfort of flatulence. Dill also can be beneficial for insomnia (go ahead, try it for the promise of shut-eye). It could be due to its polyphenols, flavonoids, and tannins, which may provide a calming effect. Some herbalists claim dill can help cure a bout of hiccups (a temporary contraction of the diaphragm). Dill is supposed to stimulate the vagus nerve (one of the most important nerves in the body), stopping a HIC-UP, HIC-UP. Note to self: Make a cup of dill tea. Use 2 teaspoons whole dill, pour in hot water, steep, and drink.

Some research (lab rats) shows dill extract may help lower insulin levels in diabetes. More research is needed. Also, dill, thanks to its myriad of antioxidants, may help enhance the immune system—something we all can use year-round.

Safety Sound Bite: Avoid dill if pregnant since it may cause miscarriage.

Shake It Up Now! Dill has been beneficial for centuries for its medicinal advantages, but it is also beneficial for culinary usage. I have dried dill leaves also called dill weed (which are mild) in a jar on a spice rack; and I do favor fresh dill for salads in summertime. It is available both whole and ground. Dill is versatile and can be used in salads, vegetables, and breads. Dill is used in tea, too. You can brew a cup of the herb and strain it or purchase tea bags online or at a health food store.

Anti-Stressing

Dill-Lemon Potato Salad

Potato salad and I go way back. My mom's old-fashioned egg potato salad is my go-to favorite. And of course, the herb-a-licious dill-infused variety at the river. Once I settled down again to return to college, one evening I whipped up a batch of potato salad for friends. In hindsight, the chunky salad was boring like a stale day-old buy at the deli. No texture, no aroma, no taste. I blame it on no herbs or spices in my minimalist kitchen for a graduate student. Perhaps that's why it ended up staying a mound in the serving bowl. Here is my new, herby version of potato salad, and there is a burst of flavor in every bite.

3 pounds russet potatoes or new potatoes, unpeeled,
*   cooked, and quartered*
¼ cup red onion, chopped
½ cup celery, chopped
2 hardboiled eggs, chopped
¾ cup store-bought mayonnaise with infused olive oil
2 tablespoons fresh or dried dill
2 tablespoons fresh for dried chives
Sea salt to taste
Lemon black pepper to taste (Mountain Rose Herbs)
Thyme sprigs for garnish

In a pan, cover potatoes with water and boil until tender. Remove from stovetop. Cool. Cut potatoes into quarters or cubes. Put potatoes into a large mixing bowl. Add onion, celery, and eggs. Mix in mayonnaise but keep the salad chunky. Add dill, chives, salt, and pepper. Chill for at least 2 hours. Garnish with thyme sprigs.

Serves 10 to 12.

Done with dill. It's time to meet and greet a comeback herb that may be or should be in your kitchen cabinet. You may have watched TV celeb chefs use fennel in recipes. Fennel—dried or fresh—gets its day in the kitchen in the next chapter.

HEALING HIGHLIGHTS FROM NATURE'S GARDEN-FEST

✓ Dill goes back to ancient times in the Mediterranean and has a history of being used by well-known historical people.

✓ Today, we know dill has plenty of antidepressant properties in it to make it a superherb providing mood boosting powers for you to savor in present-day for work-life balance.

✓ Teach your children well . . . add dill to dishes—not just pickles— because this herb can help guard against obesity, heart disease, and diabetes.

✓ Adding dill to your herb collection and a plant-based diet is a trend that is here to stay; it can help keep boomers and even their parents living longer as well as younger generations.

✓ In four words—dill helps tummy trouble. If you or yours are coping with a bout of stomach woes, dill can come to the rescue.

✓ Include dill in a spicy dish, vegetable salad, or even tea to get its multiple health benefits.

Fennel

(Umbelliferae)

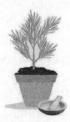

*There's fennel for you, and columbines. There's rue for
you; and here's some for me. We may call it herb of
grace o' Sundays.*
—WILLIAM SHAKESPEARE, *Hamlet* (1527–1610)

In my college days, I learned the art of utilizing fennel, an Italian herb
with a licorice-like taste. A fellow classmate and waitressing co-worker
invited me to hitchhike with her to Alaska—a state where she told me
self-reliance, a hardy life, and herbs like dried fennel seeds get you
through the harsh winters.

One day at work I shared my angst about my stomach sounds.
Drinking carbonated beverages and chewing bubble gum was causing
tummy trouble. "Have you tried fennel tea?" she asked. "My mother
and grandmother in Homer use the herb for good digestion."

That night I strained the fennel seeds she gave to me for brewing a cup of tea. It worked! Soon, my friend traveled North away from the Lower Forty-Eight, to enjoy nature—and fennel seeds. I paired juicy figs plucked from the trees nearby college and work; and sipped fennel tea—a reminder of my friend in Alaska.

THE FAMILY TREE OF FENNEL

The roots of this hardy herb with yellow flowers and feathery leaves are found in southern Europe, Australia, and North America, according to the Herb Society of America. What's more, the society points out that all the parts, including the bulb, flowers, leaves, pollen, seeds, and stalk, of the fennel plant can be eaten. In fact, fennel was put to work in interesting ways in ancient times.

"Fennel was used by ancient Egyptians as food and medicine," notes HSA. "It has been reported that fennel was used as a snake bite remedy in ancient China." Interestingly, fennel was also touted as the stamina-inducing herb for marathon warriors.

Fennel, the Herb for Champions

As the popular legend goes, the HSA explains, fennel is linked to the beginning of the marathon, a longwinded race. Historians report back in 490 B.C., amazingly, an Athenian messenger named Pheidippides carried a fennel stalk on his 150-mile two-day marathon to Sparta. It was his mission to deliver the news of the great victory over Persia in the Battle of Marathon. It has been reported that the combat was fought in a field of wild fennel.

FENNEL PLANT POWER: SURPRISE STUFF

The fennel bulb is rich in phytonutrients, which are key to its healing powers. It contains anethole and estragole (antibacterial compounds that kill germs). Fennel has flavonoids such as quercetin and apigenin, antioxidants that provide antibacterial and anti-inflammatory benefits. It also boasts terpenes fenchone and limonene, which help wounds to heal.[1]

One raw fennel bulb, according to the USDA Nutrient Database, contains 73 calories, 2.9 grams of protein, no cholesterol, 7.3 grams of dietary fiber, 360 milligrams of potassium, and other essential nutrients. Fennel is also a good source of antioxidant vitamins A and C, B vitamins, calcium, and iron.[2]

GROUNDBREAKING DISCOVERIES

Fennel is a heart-healthy herb because of its nutrients. The calcium, potassium, and magnesium all can help lower blood pressure, and this in turn helps guard your heart from working overtime, so to speak. Also, fennel contains nitrates and these little guys have vasodilatory properties, which means they, like minerals, keep your blood pressure numbers healthier.

Yes, life comes with stressors that can hike blood pressure. Relieving symptoms of depression and anxiety when events get hectic can be done. Fennel may help you to deal, say researchers. Researchers conducted a study at Mashhad University of Medical Science in Iran, providing 100 milligrams of fennel in soft capsules twice daily for two months to sixty postmenopausal women. The results: Fennel has phytoestrogenic properties that may be helpful without side effects. There was borderline and significant improvement. Further research is needed to pinpoint the reasons why the herb can act like an antidepressant pill. While the verdict is still out, it certainly couldn't hurt to add fennel to your diet or a cup of tea.[3]

Did someone say fennel is cancer-fighting? It may be. Its selenium is a mineral that can help prevent inflammation and decrease tumor growth. Its dietary fiber (found in fruits, vegetables, and whole grains) are heart-healthy and may lower the risk of developing colorectal cancer, too.

Bountiful Benefits: Not unlike anise, fennel is flavored for its usefulness! It can stave off heartburn and alleviate gas. Fennel tea is not uncommon and used for its help with digestive problems, including flatulence. The tea version of fennel with its antibacterial compounds also can be helpful when applied topically to remedy strained eye problems, by using compresses on the eyelids. But both fennel seeds and leaves are used, too.

Shake It Up Now! Essential oils from seeds of fennel are often added in cosmetics, perfume, soaps, and pharmaceuticals. Its bulbs are used as flavorings in baked goods, cooking, desserts, and Mediterranean herb blends such as my favorite herbes de Provence. It is available in fresh and dried form at the grocery store and online.

Digestion-Regulating

Stuffed Figs with Fennel Seeds

Figs and fennel seeds are a gift from nature. I love figs (off the tree not dried in a ring, which I can attest may chip a tooth) and fennel. One fiber-rich fig and fennel seeds can help you loosen up at any age. Try this recipe, inspired by my central Californian cooking mentor, Gemma Sciabica. We both know what it's like to eat fresh fruit off the tree and the power of fennel seeds.

1 pound white or dark dried moist figs
1 cup confectioners sugar
2 tablespoons fennel seeds
⅓ cup rum, anisette, Galliano or Strega liqueur
(optional)
6 bay leaves

Trim off stems, cut figs open down on one side lengthwise. Place 1 or 2 almonds in each fig, press them shut again. In container, place a layer of stuffed figs. Sprinkle with some fennel seeds, sugar, liqueur, and place 2 bay leaves on top. Continue layering figs, seeds, sugar, liqueur, and bay leaves. Cover with foil, keep refrigerated. Keeps for months, longer in a freezer.

Makes 1 pound.

(Courtesy: Gemma Sanita Sciabica, *Cooking with California Olive Oil: Treasured Family Recipes*)

Now that I've taken dill off the table, the next herb is one that is most likely familiar to you and vampires. Let's take an up-close look at garlic and all of its remarkable healing virtues.

HEALING HIGHLIGHTS FROM NATURE'S GARDEN-FEST

✓ Make fennel part of your diet because it's got anti-inflammatory benefits that can help you at any age, whether you're coping with pain of PMS, IBS, or arthritis aches.

✓ Fennel is one herb to help you stave off a bout of the blues or even minor depression.

✓ Got irregularity on your mind? Improve your plumbing with fennel tea! That's what herbalists will tell you, and your stomach bloating and flatulence may be history.

✓ Take fennel, like, as needed. Include it in a salad, vegetables, or use your imagination.

✓ Skip the salt, an overused spice that can spike blood pressure. That's where herbs like fennel come into play. SUBSTITUTE fennel for salt.

Garlic

(Liliaceae)

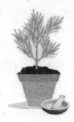

What garlic is to food, insanity is to art.
—AUGUSTUS SAINT-GAUDENS

As a thirty-ish graduate and health gastronome, living in the San Francisco Bay Area, I escaped south to the Gilroy Garlic Festival for the thrill of it. The annual event was crowded, garlic aroma filled the hot summer air. The garlic-centric scents permeated a different smell in each food booth. There were so many stands filled with so many garlic foods to sample and buy. I, of course, did both.

I ended up munching on garlicky onion rings. I relished a slice of sizzling garlic and basil vegetarian pizza, followed by a garlic cold and creamy ice cream cone. I brought home a bag of garlic bulbs to spice up my rice and vegetable dinners—my staples for losing body fat and gaining muscle. Not to forget a ceramic garlic braid I valued and hung in the kitchen as a reminder of how I lived near the garlic capital of the nation. And whenever I get the craving to visit the Pacific Ocean, a visit to Gilroy for fresh garlic bulbs is on the to-do list each and every time for the sensory thrill of it.

THE FAMILY TREE OF GARLIC

Food historians report six thousand years ago, garlic was recognized. Romans and Greeks believed garlic was ideal for stamina—and people in the Middle Ages needed vim and vigor to cope with a hardy lifestyle. Garlic was one of known herbs used to guard against the bubonic plagues.

Hippocrates, a Greek doctor and the father of modern medicine, is believed to have used garlic for curing both infections and sprains.

During the Victorian era, the herb was believed to be strong and too bitter to enjoy. Also, some herbalists claim religious groups, such as Buddhists, stayed clear of the harsh herb. In fact, garlic was believed to have aphrodisiac properties and was forbidden to eat by some people.

In 1990, the First World Congress on Garlic was held in Washington D.C., the place where it was noted that garlic was acknowledged as a scientifically supported healing herb.

A Farmer's Ode to a Garlic Farm

Finding an organic garlic farmer to teach me what goes down on a farm wasn't too difficult. Fate brought me to a woman based in charming Yellow Springs, Ohio, not California where I thought it would be. Read on—it was Joanne who told me the story of her farm's history. Here it is, just as she wrote it . . .

In October of 2010 we planted our first garlic crop of 309 cloves, in our large backyard garden in our small southern Ohio town. That winter, I literally lost sleep worrying if the garlic would make it until spring, but spring arrived and up came the garlic. In July we plucked the bulbs from the ground one at a time, excited like it was Christmas. The colors and sizes were all so different.

After the bulbs cured, I used them in so many dishes but one evening we had friends over, and I made a very garlicky guacamole using a large purple bulb. I used my rasp to grate the garlic very fine. I must have used nearly five large cloves. The flavor was so fresh and different from anything purchased from a store. Our friends dove in eating with gusto and our neighbor exclaimed, "Oh baby, that's so good. Where did you get this?" I said, "I made it! I used the garlic we grew." Everyone clapped, laughed, and kept eating. From that minute on, I knew our farm was born. Today we plant eighty thousand cloves at each planting.

The Past: I have long been enamored with the soil of the earth, its feel between my fingers and its pleasant smell that calms me. I can remember being a small child and weeding in the garden and eating fresh vegetables just picked for dinner. I was raised in the sixties and believe my mother was ahead of her time as we ate fresh naturally grown produce. So, it was just natural that I sought land many years ago where I could start my own garden, which was large enough to feed a few families. It was always my dream to farm, so I made that happen.

I was simply in love with garlic and all its varieties and different flavors, uses, and even its viability and health benefits. I truly believe it is the medicine of life. I can't remember a time that I didn't cook with fresh garlic. Sure, you can use the powdered form but there is nothing like a bulb being pulled from the earth and using it fresh or letting it cure and deepen to its full flavor.

Turban varieties are my favorite early summer garlic to use right from the ground. The bulb is fat and squatty with large cloves that perch in a manner to give it the shape of a turban. It's a true summer experience I look forward to at harvest time to make a fresh colorful salad. I usually grate several cloves on harvest day and blend it with a light olive oil, a pinch of salt, grind of pepper, a slosh of red wine vinegar or a squeeze of half a lemon, or both, and pour it over fresh sliced garden-grown Black Krim tomatoes mixed with young lettuce, torn fresh basil, fresh young corn cut right off its stalk, and some crisp cool cucumber and red onion just before serving. Sometimes I'll add kalamata olives and a toss of feta cheese. I plan this meal around harvest, which for us is late June to early July.

The Present: Our farm is situated in Ohio where we grow over forty varieties of hard neck and soft neck garlic and sell our garlic seed across the United States to farmers, CSAs, gardeners, and anyone wanting to grow and eat garlic. Recently we had a customer fly in on his own plane and land in a nearby field to pick up his garlic. I tried to keep myself calm and reserve my giggles for later. It was a real treat. I think it is the sharing of life with those that I meet that makes farming so rewarding for me. Each season I tell my customers they are the reason I do this. For more information, you can find us at www.madrivergarlic-growers.com.

GARLIC PLANT POWER: SURPRISE STUFF

Essential compounds in garlic are well, essential. One important ingredient from garlic is allicin, a heart-healthy treasure that's also found in the other vegetable—onion. Another compound worth noting is diallyl disulfide, which is in the anti-cancer lock box. Its plentiful list of ingredients makes this herb antimicrobial, anti-viral, heart-healthy, and a cancer fighter tool.

Garlic may not make the grade as a super nutrient-dense herb. But that does not mean antioxidant-rich garlic is unhealthy! Like vinegar and olive oil, remarkable garlic deserves its own book! Here, take a glance at about three-and-a-half ounces of garlic, from the United States Department of Agriculture: Water, 61 percent; carbohydrate, 30.8 grams; protein, 6.2 grams; dietary fiber, 1.5 grams; fat, 0.2 grams; potassium, 259 milligrams; phosphorus, 202 milligrams; calcium, 29 milligrams; sodium, 19 milligrams; iron, 1.5 milligrams; and ascorbic acid, 15 milligrams.

GROUNDBREAKING DISCOVERIES

Garlic is known as the heart-healthy herb, thanks to its compounds, especially sulfur. Stacks of studies, past and present, show it can help keep the numbers in check for blood pressure, cholesterol, and lower the odds of heart attacks and strokes.

Also, heart-healthy garlic is an immune system booster, which can lower your risk of developing cancer. University of Buffalo and the University of Puerto Rico researchers say that garlic and onion may reduce the odds of developing breast cancer by 67 percent. Lead researcher Gauri Desai pointed out that Puerto Rico has lower breast cancer numbers, compared to America. In the journal *Nutrition and Cancer*, he emphasized women in Puerto Rico consume more garlic and onion, two ingredients in the condiment sofrito, which is used in bean and rice dishes.[1]

Not to ignore garlic and its ability to keep your blood sugar levels steady so diabetes doesn't enter your life. Past research has shown that "garlic aided the liver to pull sugar out of the blood and encouraged the pancreas to make more insulin." This, in turn, may be able to get blood sugar to a steady range.[2]

Bountiful Benefits: Many people I know use garlic for its medicinal benefits. Take Robert, a sixty-ish poet who wrote for literary magazines. He was a devout garlic lover. When I visited him in the afternoon, the scent of garlic led me into the kitchen. He was there every day chopping fresh garlic cloves, which are used for both medicinal and culinary healing powers. He passionately added the herb to pastas, salads, seafood, and vegetables. He believed that a raw clove of garlic would keep his heart young and body cancer-free. "I eat it raw," he said, munching on a small chunk of the white herb, "but also sauté it in my food for health benefits."

Holistic doctors believe in the healing powers of garlic, too. Herbal expert Alan Keith Tillotson, R.H., Lac, Ph.D., of Chrysalis Natural Medicine Clinic, Wilmington, Delaware, told me: "I personally use fresh garlic almost every day on my raw salad. I take extra if traveling in closed spaces like airplanes—in that case I use a garlic capsule." And that takes us full circle because it is known that garlic contains antiviral compounds.

Shake It Up Now: Garlic is a popular culinary herb in a variety of dishes. My personal favorite is sautéing the cloves to give it a mellow flavor in stir-fries and herby Italian sauces. I eat garlic when I am traveling. One trip to Seattle on the night before flying home, I felt a cold coming on. I ordered artisan vegetarian garlic pasta. I sipped herbal tea while savoring bits of garlic, tomatoes, and olives. I scheduled my flight later to get a good night's sleep. I did not get sick and I give credit to the garlic, nature's cure that protected me like it may have done in the Middle Ages when people used it to fight the bubonic plague.

Interestingly, black garlic (it has been aged) is a trend in the twenty-first century. It is known to be used in Asian cuisine and is touted for its heart-healthy benefits. Black garlic is used in pasta to pizza, and is available online and at health food stores. Garlic is available in many forms, from chopped fresh cloves to minced, ground powder, and in spice blends. Capsules contain the active ingredient allicin. It can be consumed and used topically.

Safety Sound Bite: Do not consume more than two cloves of raw garlic daily. If you overindulge, the consequences can be digestive problems, such as heartburn or acid reflux, and flatulence. Remember, less is more.

Anti-Viral-Enhancing

Pasta with Garlic and Tomatoes

❖ ❖ ❖

Pasta with garlic and tomatoes is an Italian dish that can be made quickly. Make sure to use your favorite extra virgin olive oil for it. This recipe is easy on the budget. Two favorite herbs—garlic and parsley—make it a perfect dish for any time year-round. It is a fail-proof recipe that can be used for a side dish or a light meal.

¾ pound of spaghetti, cooked
Sea salt to taste
6 tablespoons extra virgin olive oil
8 garlic cloves, minced
¾ teaspoon lemon pepper
1 cup Roma tomatoes, chopped
½ cup Parm cheese, grated
Marjoram or basil for garnish

Bring a large pot of water to boil. Add pasta and salt. (Italian chefs recommend salting the water to the salinity of sea water.) Cook pasta, several minutes, until al dente (not overcooked). Drain. Do not rinse. Heat oil in a non-stick skillet over low heat, then add garlic and sauté, do not overcook. Add lemon pepper. Stir-fry tomatoes in same pan. Transfer drained pasta to warm serving bowl. Add the garlic and tomatoes to pasta. Toss. Top with cheese and garnish with marjoram or basil.

Makes 4 servings.

Next up is marjoram, an herb you may not have been acquainted with yet. Open your eyes and mind to an ancient herb that deserves to be noticed and appreciated!

HEALING HIGHLIGHTS FROM NATURE'S GARDEN-FEST

✓ Garlic has been appreciated for more than five thousand years. Sure, its origin goes back to Asia, but it was also cultivated and used in ancient Europe.

✓ This Mediterranean herb contains a mega amount of antioxidants, which provide more health benefits than its vitamins and minerals.

✓ Not only is garlic heart-healthy due to its disease-fighting compounds, it also has immune-enhancing properties . . .

✓ . . . It's these ingredients such as allicin in garlic that may help to guard against viral infections, including colds and flu.

✓ Garlic can be consumed raw or cooked and enjoyed for its aroma, flavor, and health benefits . . .

✓ Ask everyday people what their favorite edible herb is and more than likely garlic will be on the top of their must-have list— including mine!

✓ . . . But amazingly, garlic is also used topically, which provides many benefits to help heal skin infections and inflammation.

Marjoram

(Lamiaceae)

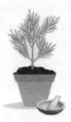

*Hot lavender, mints, savory, marjoram; The marigold,
that goes to bed wi' the sun, and with him rise weeping.*
—WILLIAM SHAKESPEARE, *The Winter's Tale* (1610-1) act 4

Garlic pairs well with marjoram—like peanut butter and jam. After the Gilroy Garlic Festival, I met a charismatic chef's helper. We were both gourmands living in the San Francisco Bay Area. We loved pizza with garlic. One Indian summer weekend in San Carlos my friend brought me the gift of fresh marjoram from his small garden. The herb looked like a hybrid of fresh oregano and basil leaves. We used garlic and marjoram on our homemade pizza with ripe tomatoes from my plants on the back porch. It was a fragrant, flavorful feast we shared in my rustic Mediterranean-style bungalow. These days, when I make pizza it takes me back to the romantic herb marjoram, like the allure and novelty of a blossoming romance.

THE FAMILY TREE OF MARJORAM

Let me introduce you to the plant that comes from North Africa. It is also known as French marjoram, wild marjoram—and sweet marjoram, on the authority of the Herb Society of America, "is sweeter than oregano," which is actually in the same family. Marjoram often is confused with spicy oregano but they have different healing powers. Marjoram goes back centuries when it was appreciated for its many virtues. Historians will tell you it was favored by Aphrodite, the mythical goddess. Herbal historians also note Egyptians put the herb to use as a disinfectant.

Marjoram leaves were symbolic of love (it's ironic I discovered this tidbit after my relationship ended) for newlyweds in the Middle Ages. In the time of Hippocrates, the doctor was believed to enjoy its antiseptic benefits. He was hardly alone. The herb is noted to be used for respiratory ailments as well as keeping foods fresh long ago. Nowadays, marjoram graces the hillsides in Mediterranean countries, North America, and Western Asia.

Marjoram, Mountain of Joy

Herbal historians tell the legend of marjoram, the Mediterranean herb that was dubbed "mountain of joy." It is believed marjoram adopted its sweet and satisfying aroma when handled by Venus, the Roman goddess of love, beauty, desire, and even prosperity. Perhaps it was her touch that gave the herb its ability to be helpful in warranting a long and rewarding life rich in happiness.

MARJORAM PLANT POWER: SURPRISE STUFF

This herbal wonder contains anti-inflammatory compounds that can be beneficial for many ailments creating discomfort with aches and pains. It contains antibacterial, antifungal, and antiseptic properties. This, in result, means marjoram can fight germs and viruses. Marjoram is also praised for its anti-spasmodic powers, which can be helpful with the nervous system and female woes, like pre-menstrual cramps. Not to ignore it is rich in polyphenols, which are natural disease-fighting antioxidants, including carvacrol, luetin, and zeaxan-thin.

Marjoram is a nutrient-rich herb that deserves more recognition. It's chock-full of disease-fighting antioxidants, including vitamin A, vitamin C, and beta carotene. Also, this Mediterranean wellness herb gives you an amazing amount of blood-clotting vitamin K. Not to forget it is packed with essential minerals, like bone-boosting calcium, copper, iron, magnesium, manganese, and potassium.

GROUNDBREAKING DISCOVERIES

Antioxidant-rich marjoram can help your heart stay healthy. This Mediterranean herb has the amazing ability to relax and widen the blood vessels, which helps keep blood pressure levels at healthy numbers (120/80 or a bit lower). The delicate scent of marjoram can also calm the nervous system, and that is good for the heart, too.

The healing powers of today's unsung heroic herb marjoram are plentiful. It is still used as an aid for respiratory ailments, including bronchitis, colds, and flu. Its extracts can guard against fungi and bacteria. Today, in the twenty-first century, germs, viruses, and superbugs are lurking everywhere, in your workplace, when on a plane, or even in your home! Antimicrobial marjoram may help bolster your immune system so you will be resistant to an infectious bug or even a superbug that is resistant to antibiotics.

Enter the novel coronavirus of 2019–20. The outbreak of the respiratory illness also called COVID-19 developed into a challenging pandemic affecting the health and well-being of people—all ages—around the globe. The coronavirus wreaks havoc on your immune system. Medical doctors advise guarding your body with a nutrient-dense diet. That's where superherbs, like marjoram paired with other antioxidant-rich herbs and spices and superfoods come into play. Health experts believe vitamins D and C and other nutrients found in herbs in spices may guard against deadly flu and superbugs – and help your body fight a respiratory illness, too.

Researchers have discovered and pinpointed plant essential oils found in marjoram, like other Mediterranean plants, which have anti-inflammatory and anti-cancer properties. This, in result, means including the herb in a healthy diet and lifestyle, used in your diet food and even a tea, may help to lower your odds of developing cancer.[1]

Bountiful Benefits: The herb can also be beneficial in quelling tummy woes, such as gas and indigestion. Thanks to its anti-inflammatory compounds, marjoram is used to soothe pain. It may help quell a throbbing tension headache or pesky backache. It truly is under appreciated in the twenty-first century and is making a comeback as a versatile home cure remedy.

Shake It Up Now! Marjoram is used in the perfume industry, notes the HSA, to scent cologne, lotions, and soaps. It is also a culinary herb used in savory dishes. Marjoram is available fresh at grocery stores and farmers' markets. Also, dried form is available at grocery stores, health food stores, and online. When I use its fresh organic leaves (available in the produce aisle in a rectangular plastic container at the supermarket) and combine it with garlic, bittersweet memories of the "love" pizza visit me. Dried marjoram is in my spice cabinet. It can be enjoyed year-round in teas and with fresh seasonal fruits. Marjoram is also used in a home garden and aromatherapy indoors.

Mediterranean Oven-Baked Garlic and Marjoram Pizza

❖ ❖ ❖

Did you know pizza topped with marjoram is a superfood? It can be super good for you if you use whole grain crust, tomatoes, olives, olive oil, and spinach, all are foods in the heart-healthy Mediterranean diet.

1 store-bought pre-baked whole wheat pizza crust
    (Boboli)
½ cup marinara sauce, organic infused with olive oil
1 cup feta cheese, crumbled or mozzarella

½ cup Roma tomatoes, chopped
¼ cup mushrooms
½ cup spinach, fresh
1 clove garlic, minced
½ teaspoon oregano
1 tablespoon marjoram leaves

Preheat the oven to 350 degrees F. Place crust on a nonstick pan. Spread with sauce. Sprinkle cheese over sauce. Top with tomatoes, mushrooms, spinach, and garlic. Sprinkle with oregano and marjoram. Bake for approximately 20 to 30 minutes until crust is light golden brown and cheese is bubbly.

Serves 4.

So now that I've put another versatile herb into your growing collection, it's time to bring to you another spicy wonder. Most likely, you're familiar with nutmeg, celebrated during the end-of-the-year holiday season—but it has so much to offer it should be enjoyed year-round. Find out why in the next chapter.

HEALING HIGHLIGHTS FROM NATURE'S GARDEN-FEST

✓ Marjoram, a European herb, goes way back in time to being used in the Mediterranean countries, mythology, and appreciated by its diverse peoples.
✓ This herb is healing for you and your tribe. Marjoram can do a body and mind good with its antioxidants, antimicrobial, anti-inflammatory compounds.
✓ Dried or fresh, marjoram is an herb to mix and match with other herbs since it is healing and worthy of incorporating into your diet regime and lifestyle.
✓ This Mediterranean herb can help enhance good digestion and

even lower the risk of you developing cancer. Note to self: Nobody is immune.

✓ Marjoram is nature's mood-boosting herb that is worth trying, especially if you're prone to blanket cocooning during the winter blues or spring doldrums.

✓ Marjoram is versatile in cooking but it has other uses, from home remedies to usefulness in the outdoors.

Nutmeg

(Myristicaceae)

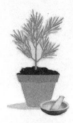

He's of the colour of the nutmeg. And of the heat
of the ginger.
—WILLIAM SHAKESPEARE, *Second Tetraology in Plain and*
Simple English

Sitting around a white flocked Christmas tree, in my childhood I
sipped eggnog sprinkled with brown specks of nutmeg on top. While
anticipating opening one present for the evening it is the feel-good
holiday spicy beverage that revisited me decades later . . . One late fall
morning in Seattle, Washington, in a hotel room overlooking Puget
Sound, I ordered breakfast: French toast with artisan bread, and nutmeg. The aromatic spice was a blast from the past—nature's gift of
home. I anticipated to be back inside my Tahoe cabin, surrounded by
pine trees shrouded with snow, family, my dog—and eggnog with a
dash of fresh nutmeg.

THE FAMILY TREE OF NUTMEG

The roots of nutmeg are intriguing. It is the seed, not a nut, of an evergreen tree (like cardamom), the ones that grow in Indonesia, the place where the Portuguese discovered it in the sixteenth century. Food historians say the Dutch and British both wanted nutmeg, and eventually ended up controlling the nutmeg trade, restructuring the workers at the plantations.

Culinary historian Michael Krondl in the 1600s, note historians, knew nutmeg had a huge following because of its versatility as a culinary spice and healing powers. Nutmeg was also one of the common spices to help prevent contracting the deadly black plague.

During World War II (before I was born but my parents shared stories of their experiences), Wartime Cake was popular and printed in a 1942 Betty Crocker booklet of wartime recipes. The cake included both spicy cloves and nutmeg.

NUTMEG PLANT POWER: SURPRISE STUFF

Nutmeg is so much more than a spice to sprinkle on holiday eggnog. According to the USDA Nutrient Database, essential ingredients include copper, dietary fiber, folate, macelignan, manganese, thiamine, and vitamin B6. But you won't be eating nutmeg by the spoonful. However, its other components are the real thing that can give you the real results.

Nutmeg contains antibacterial and anti-inflammatory compounds. This warming spice contains antioxidant power, including plant pigments like cyanidins, essential oils, such as phenylpropanoids and terpenes, and phenol compounds—protocatechuic, ferulic, and caffeic acids. It contains a compound called myristicin which can enhance memory. Macelignan, myristic acid, and trimyristin are antibacterial properties.[1]

GROUNDBREAKING DISCOVERIES

Worldwide, cancer incidence continues to skyrocket—and studies show that natural remedies could cut your risk. Myristicin in nutmeg may prevent growth of cancer cells. suggests research in the journal *Chemo-Biological Interactions*. The researchers explain the compound from the spice regulates genes of the DNA damage response pathways in human cancer cells.[2]

Alcohol, obesity, prescription drugs, and viruses can cause harm to your liver, a vital organ to detoxify chemical in the body. But Chinese researchers say myrislignan, the compound in found in nutmeg, protects against liver damage.[3]

Bountiful Benefits: Sleepless nights affect all of us sooner or later. Nutmeg may help to get shut-eye whether you're in Seattle or New York. The warm spice can also help guard against asthma, stomach pain, and is a kidney detoxifier. It may dissolve kidney stones (a friend of mine coped with this painful ailment) and kidney infections.

Safety Sound Bite: No more than one tablespoon of nutmeg per day is recommended.

Shake It Up Now! Nutmeg, a popular holiday spice that is used in pies and puddings, custard, and eggnog—a favorite of mine. I use a premium organic brand, sometimes low-fat, other times I splurge. Nutmeg can be used in ground form but it is also available whole and fresh grated from the nut. It is used in both Indian cuisine and French cuisine such as egg and cheese dishes. This warm spicy flavor is also often found in blends. Freshly grated nutmeg from the nut (like dark chocolate) is preferred to be used by sophisticated chefs. Whole and ground nutmeg is found in supermarkets.

Anti-Inflammatory

French Toast

French toast is a staple breakfast that goes back in time. In the twentieth century, my mom would use white bread, egg, whole milk, and nondescript syrup. I use whole grain bread, low-fat organic milk, and Canadian maple syrup rich in antioxidants. This version (yes, do use the good syrup from Vermont or Quebec) is different and delicious because of both the citrus and nutmeg twist.

8 eggs
1 cup orange juice
2 cups milk
1 teaspoon freshly ground cinnamon
1 teaspoon freshly ground nutmeg
1 tablespoon vanilla extract
16 slices Challah bread [a special bread in Jewish
*   cuisine often braided] or another medium density,*
*   slightly sweet bread*
2 tablespoon unsalted butter, melted

In a large bowl, combine the eggs, orange juice, milk, cinnamon, nutmeg, and vanilla and whisk until well blended. Dip the bread in the egg batter and allow it to absorb some of the liquid. Heat the butter in a large sauté pan over medium-high heat and cook slices of bread until golden brown. Serve while hot with maple syrup, apple butter, jam, or preserves.

Yields 8.

(Courtesy: Chef Ann Foundation)

Back to the Mediterranean we go to understand the history and healing powers behind an herb. You've probably tasted this fragrant herb in Italian cuisine, as I have done. Does oregano resonate with your desire for Italian herbs? If not, it may do just that after you find out all the good things about its advantages. Read on.

Healing Highlights from Nature's Garden-Fest

✓ Ah, nutmeg, a holiday popular spice savored in eggnog and pumpkin pie has so much more to offer year-round as a spice.

✓ It is believed nutmeg can enhance memory thanks to its myristicin compound, which can be helpful. Yeah, nutmeg can guard against a senior pause or delayed recall during multi-tasking which can make anyone forget a simple name or event.

✓ The don'ts include don't limit nutmeg to eggnog and custard. IT IS so much more! ...

✓ ... Include nutmeg in your diet year-round. Top it on soups, vegetables, sweet potato pie, and even a pasta salad!

✓ But hold the shaker, sprinkle s-l-o-w-l-y because a little will suffice for health's sake. Too much is not better.

Oregano

(*Lamiaceae*)

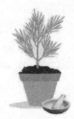

*Praised be You, my Lord, through our Sister, Mother
Earth, who sustains and governs us, producing varied
fruits with coloured flowers and herbs.*
—FRANCIS OF ASSISI

Oregano is an herb dotted in dishes served in my home, past and present. My dad, a widower in his seventies, planned a home-cooked fish dinner with his new girlfriend and me for a grad school gift. I planned movies; she brought food—five courses. I was surprised. Her epicurean cooking with familiar oregano—like my mom used...She served Lobster Oreganata, which is a split lobster topped with breadcrumbs, seasoned with oregano. It was a night of comfort like back in childhood. The gift of the familiar oregano aroma and flavor reconnected me to my mom's spirit *and* bonded us—my new surrogate mom. Whenever I smell oregano it links me to my dad—and two mothers.

THE FAMILY TREE OF OREGANO

The roots of oregano come from the Mediterranean countries, including Greece, Italy, and Turkey. Its leaves are the parts used. Sure, oregano is linked to Italian cuisine, and this herb has roots back to 3000 B.C.

The consensus of historians is that both the Greeks and Romans appreciated oregano. Since the herb grew in the mountains of the Mediterranean the Greeks called it "Mountain Joy." The love for oregano increased and was used in all of Europe.

Once World War II was over, thanks to soldiers in Europe, the herb came to America because the GIs enjoyed the flavor in Italian food. In the last half of the twentieth century, oregano was used in Italian cuisine. In the fifties and sixties, I recall the aromatic spice was sprinkled in my family's spaghetti, ravioli, soups, and stews to give it that flavorful panache.

A Love Story with Oregano and Marjoram

As historians tell it, Aphrodite, the Greek goddess of the herbal pair, oregano and marjoram is connected to happiness. The story goes like this. The mythical woman cultivated the herb in a garden on top of Mount Olympus. Her mission was to let flatlanders see what joy brings to mind. Marjoram was to have the aroma of the goddess on it. And this way, any human could inhale the aromatic herb, any time. Aphrodite, known as the goddess of love, had plant passion and was connected to love and marriage. It is believed couples would wear crowns made of oregano and marjoram on their wedding nights with dreams of reaping the rewards of a fruitful marriage.

OREGANO PLANT POWER: SURPRISE STUFF

The amount of the chemical carvacrol (a creosote-scented phenol) and thymol in oregano provides antibacterial, anti-fungal, and anti-viral benefits. Ask any antioxidant researcher and they will tell you oregano may be one of the superherbs with the most antioxidants.

Refer to the ORAC chart in chapter 1. Oregano and cloves appear to contain the highest antioxidant activity. Bring on the marinara sauce with oregano for sauces to pizza.

Oregano provides a nutritional bonanza of vitamins and minerals. It contains vitamin A, vitamin C, and niacin. The minerals include boron, calcium and tryptophan, copper, iron, manganese, magnesium, iron, potassium, and zinc.

GROUNDBREAKING DISCOVERIES

No, consuming oregano in a marinara sauce is not a cancer cure. But, oregano contains rosmarinic acid, which has been found to have antimutagenic and anti-carcinogenic properties. In simple English that means this multipurpose herb may help to keep your body's cells healthy and lower your odds of developing cancer.[1]

Researchers at Long Island University in New York studied carvacrol, the mighty chemical found in oregano. When it was added to cancer cells in the lab, it destroyed them. More research is needed before we can say, "Eat your Italian oregano pizza to keep your prostate healthy"—but past research shows promise.

Bountiful Benefits: Oregano is not new; it has been raved about for centuries. After all, its advantages are limitless. This "carminative" herb like oregano is praised for its antiseptic compounds that help aid colds, congestion, the flu, and sore throats. Herbalists say Hippocrates utilized oregano for respiratory ailments. The herb also is used to treat digestive ailments, such as flatulence "gas," which is uncomfortable and embarrassing if heard in public.

Shake It Up Now! As a girl, I recall seeing oregano in a McCormick's red and white can sitting on the shelf with other spices. It was sprinkled in Italian dishes, like fish, tomato-based pastas and sauces, and meats. Dried oregano is popular but fresh oregano leaves (like bay) can be used, too. Also, oil of oregano supplements are available but consult with your healthcare practitioner.

When I asked the question, "What two seasonings would you select if you were stranded on an island?" Seafarer, Mediterranean foodie expert Dr. Will Clower (who just landed in Africa by his boat) answered,

"Oregano goes with everything, and is so user-friendly," he said. "The other would be black pepper, because it is so versatile and used in everything for both spice and flavor!"

Personally, when I make a semi-homemade pizza or any Italian dish, oregano (either fresh or dried) is often used. Oregano nourishes my body because of its nutrients. But it also feeds my heart and soul because this Mediterranean herb connects me to my two mothers who fancied the art of cooking with herbs like oregano.

Cancer-Protecting

Mom's Dried Cod Roast Organata

I do cherish the memory of my past fish feasts. Also, cod contains more omega-3 fatty acids than other fish. Omega-3s help alleviate PMS symptoms and also lower cholesterol levels, lowering risk of developing heart disease. This recipe is created by my dear friend, a down-to-earth cook I respect, especially when it comes to preparing fish recipes. It includes rosemary, a woody herb, native to Mediterranean regions like France. European countries often use rosemary (and have since the middle ages). Rosemary is commonly found in Italian cooking, like this dish, with plenty of herb and spice treasures to discover. And it pairs nicely with cayenne for a bit of heat.

2 pounds dried cod, cut into serving pieces
1 onion, diced
1 cup celery, diced
2 carrots, diced
½ cup Romano cheese, grated
1 teaspoon sage or tarragon
Salt, pepper, and cayenne to taste
4 potatoes cut into wedges

1 tablespoon fresh rosemary, chopped
Oregano to taste
½ cup fresh basil or parsley, chopped
4 garlic cloves, minced
4 bay leaves
⅓ cup Marsala Olive Fruit Oil
4 cups fresh or canned tomatoes, chopped
1–1½ cups breadcrumbs
Olive oil for drizzling
¾ cup white wine or vermouth

Soak codfish in water 2 or 3 days, change water several times, keep refrigerated. Preheat the oven to 350 degrees F. In large bowl combine fish pieces (drained), onion, celery, carrots, cheese, sage, salt, pepper, cayenne, potatoes, rosemary, oregano, basil, garlic, bay leaves, and olive oil. Toss gently, place in greased deep roasting pan. Sprinkle with tomatoes and breadcrumbs. Drizzle all with olive oil. Pour in wine, cover. Bake for 1 hour or until potatoes and fish are tender. Remove bay leaves before serving.

Serves 4 to 6.

(Courtesy: Gemma Sanita Sciabica, *Cooking with California Olive Oil: Popular Recipes*)

My next pick has a history, too, but isn't as popular as oregano. Still, paprika is a spice worth words of gratitude. Let me count the variety of reasons why this unacknowledged healing spice made the cut.

HEALING HIGHLIGHTS FROM NATURE'S GARDEN-FEST

✓ Oregano is traced back in time as early as 3000 B.C. when Ancient Romans and Greeks put the treasure to work for its medicinal powers and flavor as a culinary herb.

✓ The healing powers of oregano are limitless, including compounds that can help treat respiratory and digestive disorders.

✓ Do note, oregano contains plenty of healthful nutrients to help stave off colds and flu, but it may even guard you against cancer, thanks to its potent chemical carvacrol.

✓ The Mediterranean diet includes oregano in its list of herbs since it is used in Italian cuisine.

✓ Including oregano with heart-healthy fare—not only pizza—not only adds flavor but essential nutrients year-round.

Paprika

(Solanaceae)

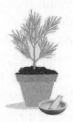

*Then fare thee well: I must go buy spices for
our sheep shearing.*
—WILLIAM SHAKESPEARE, CLOWN, *A Winter's Tale, Act IV,*
4, 2048

The first time I encountered "red gold," as Hungarians call it, was see-ing the red powder dusted on decorative deviled eggs at a picnic. The thing is, paprika is so much more than a colorful garnish. Fast-forward to Chicken Paprika and Mashed Potatoes—a dinner my mom made one winter weekend during a thunderstorm. As she served chicken and taters (both sprinkled with red specks), the power went out. In candle-light, she shared a trick of cooking with spices. She explained that when the Eastern Europe spice is heated, its mild flavor creates an extra kick to cuisine. Her wisdom and spicy chicken dish made me feel warm and fuzzy—in my comfort zone. These days, when I use paprika on French fries to garlic toast or popcorn, it is a welcomed sign that my creative mom is watching over me—smiling and giving me a warm hug like paprika can do for food.

THE FAMILY TREE OF PAPRIKA

This spice originally comes from a tropical plant in South America and it is grown in countries such as Hungary and Spain. The Herbal Society of America points out, "Paprika is made from grinding air-dried peppers from the common pepper plant, *Capsicum annuum*." What's more, the plant produces white flower that blossom the peppers that are dried and ground into powder.

No, paprika isn't the top seller of spices in America. Interestingly, though, paprika does have its place in the spice industry for its garden-variety of antioxidants (the good guys that fight cell damage caused by molecules aka free radicals).

PAPRIKA PLANT POWER: SURPRISE STUFF

Paprika contains carotenoids, an antioxidant-rich compound that may help guard against the life-threatening diseases. The reddish color in paprika that you see as a garnish on food comes from carotenoids, two compounds, capsanthin and capsorubin. Paprika also contains lutein and zeaxanthin—two compounds that can help eye health. Not to ignore it contains healing capsaicin, like found in cayenne pepper and chili peppers.

Like other spices, paprika is a dieter's friend. One tablespoon contains only 19 calories, less than 1 gram of fat, and 2 grams of dietary fiber. These nutrients are all essential if you're losing weight and body fat or are maintaining your ideal weight to feel good and stave off diseases linked to obesity.

This red powder provides vitamin C—a lot—and even more than some fruits and vegetables. It is the vitamin C that helps your body absorb iron. Speaking of iron, paprika contains 8 percent of the daily value (good news if you're a vegetarian). Paprika also contains antioxidant E, 13 percent of the daily value, and vitamin B6, 9 percent of the daily value.

GROUNDBREAKING DISCOVERIES

Is paprika heart-healthy? Herbalists agree it can help boost blood circulation, for one. But the spice also can help you keep your blood pressure numbers in check. How exactly can a red spice powder do that? Give credit to the little chemical capsaicin. It's believed that it can relax blood vessels, which can actually lower blood pressure. But that's not all . . .

Spices that are rich in antioxidants, like paprika, may help improve triglycerides and other blood lipids, report Penn State nutritionists. That means, paprika may help to guard against a build-up of the fatty plaque that can clog your arteries and lead to strokes and cardiovascular disease.[1]

More good paprika news: The compound capsanthin, a carotenoid in this spice, may spike your good cholesterol, which can help lower your risk of developing heart disease. Also, the carotenoids in this red spice may help to lower levels of low-density lipoprotein LDL, your "bad" cholesterol. More research is needed but for now adding paprika to your diet seems worth the sprinkle or two.

Paprika is also another potential cancer fighting spice, thanks to its beta carotene, carotenoids, and other antioxidants. Past research has shown people who had blood levels of these compounds were up to one third more likely to lower the risk of developing breast cancer. More research is needed before you'll see "cancer fighting" words on the nutrition label of a paprika can. But it couldn't hurt to sprinkle the red specks on garlic toast and scrambled eggs.

Bountiful Benefits: There are studies showing the power of capsaicin, which has many health benefits and is available in many forms. Capsaicin provides anti-inflammatory perks. Yes, paprika can help your aches and pains, such as joint pain. Painful joints can be caused by strains, sprains, knees, shoulders, and even age-related osteoarthritis. When eaten in foods it may increase your body's feel-good endorphins and lessen mild pain.

The variety of antioxidants and nutrients may also improve your eye health, thanks to its antioxidants vitamin E, beta carotene, lutein, and zeaxanthin. These nutrients in paprika have been pinpointed to help guard against age-related macular degeneration (AMD) and cataracts—which both can impair your sight. A girlfriend of mine suffered from early onset of AMD. I witnessed how the symptoms affected her, whereas night driving was not an option and at work she used a computer that provided large font. Her failing eyesight challenges are enough for me to include spices, like paprika, in my diet to help maintain good vision.

Shake It Up Now! Paprika offers a variety of culinary uses, mostly in appetizers and sides like bread and potatoes. This spice is also used in many spice blends. Paprika comes in sweet, smoked, and super-hot varieties. Its colors can be red, orange, and even yellow. It is found in store-bought foods that are red, like canned soups, stews, and chili. Quality paprika is available at gourmet shops, specialty markets, online, and at some grocery stores.

Rejuvenating

Mashed Sweet Potatoes with Smoked Paprika

Julia Child mastered the art of garlic–mashed potatoes. She uses all-purpose potatoes, garlic, and red pepper (cayenne) for heat. While the chef's recipe is filled with flavor, this method of another noteworthy chef puts paprika to work to please your palate, too. Pairing sweet potatoes with paprika is different and it is the popular Cal-a-Vie Health Resort who gave me this recipe.

1 pound sweet potatoes
1 teaspoon smoked paprika

1 tablespoon maple syrup
½ teaspoon kosher or sea salt
¼ cup plus 1 tablespoon orange juice

Preheat the oven to 350 degrees F. Thoroughly wash the whole sweet potato to remove any dirt. Place it on a baking sheet and roast for one hour, or until it is soft and tender all the way to the center (pierce with knife to check). Peel the sweet potato while still warm and break it up with a potato masher. Add the smoked paprika, maple syrup, salt, and orange juice and continue mashing until smooth.

Serves 4.

(Courtesy: Chef Curtis Cooke, Cal-a-Vie, Havens, Terri and John, *Beautiful Living: Cooking the Cal-A-Vie Health Spa Way*)

Next up is a favorite herb of mine, perhaps, you too. Some folks believe it is just a garnish—not so much. Come on, let me show you how I've counted the ways why parsley is under-rated.

HEALING HIGHLIGHTS FROM NATURE'S GARDEN-FEST

✓ Paprika is an under-rated spice made from dried peppers from the plant *Capsicum annuum*.
✓ This spice is antioxidant-plentiful but it also contains some B6 and iron—calming and energizing.
✓ Not to ignore its little chemical capsaicin. It's believed that it can relax blood vessels, which can actually lower blood pressure. And there's more to this heart-healthy spice!
✓ Its antioxidant powers compound capsanthin, a carotenoid in this spice, and may spike your good cholesterol, which can help keep the arteries unclogged . . .
✓ Some research shows paprika even lowers the risk of developing

some cancers—so sprinkle it on antioxidant-rich vegetables and whole grains.

✓ Enjoy your "aha" moment when you discover the little red spice sprinkles on garlic toast or mashed taters is more than just a pretty red color on golden deviled eggs for picnics.

✓ Paprika boasts flavor when heated in dishes, like soups and stews, so remember that fact instead of calling it "just a garnish" for eggs and potato salad.

Parsley

(Umbelliferae)

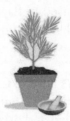

Parsley—the jewel of herbs,
both in the pot and on the plate.
—ALBERT STOCKLI

Parsley and I have a bond, thanks to Mother Nature. During my days of living in the Santa Cruz Mountains, I nurtured parsley, rosemary, and thyme in the sunny kitchen windowsills. My Labrador retriever nursed eleven pups. A hippie woman living in the woodsy town of Boulder Creek used my herb's fresh leaves for pre-menstrual symptoms. After hearing my monthly PMS complaints, she offered, and I accepted, her parsley cure challenge. The brew (and I also sprinkled the chopped herb on pasta and vegetables dishes), was a medicinal wonder. Parsley got me through bloat and dog duties, during the monthly curse. I was sold. The parsley tea cure is a woman's best friend.

The Family Tree of Parsley

Indeed, parsley has its roots in the Mediterranean regions. It was cultivated by the Greeks and the Romans in ancient days. The green herb was utilized in cooking and for its variety of medicinal powers.

As the legend goes, it was bad luck for a warrior to see the green herb before going to battle. In fact, parsley wasn't served in dishes before combat. Greek gardens were believed to include parsley, which may have spawned the phrase, "Oh! We are only at the Parsley and Rue" to show that something in progress had not come to fruition.

It is believed that Pliny noted parsley as a remedy for sick fish and also pointed out that it was used to flavor broths and sauces. During the Tudor era, parsley was believed to be a folk cure for baldness. Also, historians claim parsley was used as an antidote to guard against poisoning.

It was the *History of Plants* author, Gerard, who grew two types of parsley, flat and Curly Italian. The flat variety is tastier. The curly type, like in my fridge, is ruffled and used more as a pretty garnish.

The Legend of Parsley and Persephone

As history tells it, the god Ophletes made a connection with the queen Persephone; in Greek mythology she is the daughter of Zeus and Demeter. Persephone's husband was Hades, the god of the underworld when he died. Evidently, on the ground where his blood dried, parsley grew. It was believed Persephone's mission was to obtain and treasure Ophletes' spirit in the form of the parsley. Later, Persephone adorned memorials of the dead with parsley with the goal of gaining approval of Ophletes. It is said parsley must visit with Hades, the god of the underworld, Persephone's husband, nine times before parsley will sprout. Also, art shows Persephone carrying parsley, a symbol of her association with the God Ophletes.

PARSLEY PLANT POWER: SURPRISE STUFF

A primary compound in parsley is 1,3,8-p-menthatriene, which is in the leaves. Other key compounds are limonene and myristicin. Fresh parsley contains carotenoids lutein and zeaxanthin, too. It also boasts antioxidants vitamin C and E. But there are its nutrients to note.

Parsley contains beta-carotene, vitamin K, and vitamin B2, B3, and folic acid. Fresh parsley is a dieter's best friend. At health resort spas, nutritionists will tell you they often have parsley tea available for people who have fluid retention problems because it acts as a diuretic. The total fat content in it is almost zero. Ten sprigs of raw parsley contain 4 calories, and 1 cup has a total of 22 calories.

GROUNDBREAKING DISCOVERIES

Parsley is believed to be an anti-cancer plant food. Russian researchers from the Moscow Institute of Physics and Technology reported in the *Journal of Natural Products* superherbs, like dill and parsley (compounds extracted from parsley and dill seeds), contain cancer-fighting action. Its ability to fight cancer may be due to its antioxidants, which may prevent tumors.[1]

In addition to being an anti-cancer herb, stacks of studies prove its chlorophyll can detoxify the body. Research has shown parsley can inhibit bacterial growth in wounds, fight toxins, and stave off cell damage from cancer-causing pollutants.

Parsley Can Jump-Start Your Period!

During childbearing years, women cope with their monthly period. Plenty of women, perhaps even you, have wanted to start your period at one time or another. Hormonal imbalances, stress, and losing weight too fast are some reasons why the curse stalls instead of paying you a visit. Irregular periods can be a source of stress, too. Why? Premenstrual symptoms, such as irritability to the blues, are over the top and you just want the period to arrive. And, of course, there is the vacation or romance in your life where a period can wreak havoc on your plans, right?

Enter parsley tea. It is believed the doctor Nicholas Culpepper said, "it brings urine and women's curses" noting parsley's diuretic effect and the notion it could stave off female woes of the monthly cycle. There are two compounds, apiol and myristicin, in parsley that may stimulate blood flow in the pelvic region and uterus. Also, they may start your period.

Here's the Parsley Tea recipe: 1 tablespoon parsley, fresh leaves. Put dried root or leaves into one 8-ounce cup of boiling water. Steep parsley for about 7–8 minutes. Strain and serve with lemon and honey to taste. Repeat twice a day.

Safety Sound Bites: Avoid parsley tea if you are pregnant, or have kidney disease. Also, before starting this natural remedy, consult with your health practitioner for safety's sake.

Bountiful Benefits: Parsley is much more than a useless garnish to push to the side of your plate, like unrequited love despite what Seattle-based Susie Diamond (played by Michelle Pfeiffer) says in the "Feelings" scene of *The Fabulous Baker Boys* film. This little green cancer-fighting herb can also help keep your kidneys healthy, perhaps because it provides diuretic benefits that flush excess water in your body. I used to make a parsley tea to fight tummy bloat during premenstrual syndrome.

Shake It Up Now! Flat and curly parsley can be used dried and fresh. This herb is best served fresh, but I have a container of the dried herb and in a pinch, it does its job on a baked potato. It is available in both dried and fresh varieties at the grocery store. I've purchased it in organic form in a large bunch and inside a plastic container and in a pot, too, putting it on a shelf in the kitchen. I often thought, "If I ever travel to Alaska, I'll be sure to have parsley sprinkled on top of pasta with fresh tomatoes."

Hormonal Normalizing

Spaghetti with Olive Oil and Herbs

❖ ❖ ❖

There are a variety of ways to make pasta, a perfect side or a main dish. During the springtime through the raising puppies weeks I, like my Lab, was dog-tired. I didn't have the desire or energy to cook but needed to eat. Pasta with fresh herbs and citrus—parsley and lemon—filled me up and provided energy to keep going for the pups. This recipe is inspired by parsley, pregnancy, and PMS—and a gourmet kitchen not used enough—and to this day I have regrets about it.

14 ounces Eden whole grain spaghetti
2 tablespoons Eden Extra Virgin Olive Oil
2 teaspoons grated lemon peel (zest)
2 tablespoons lemon juice, freshly squeezed
¼ cup fresh parsley, chopped or fresh tarragon
¼ cup fresh chives, chopped fine or scallions
½ teaspoon Eden Sea Salt, or to taste
⅛ teaspoon freshly ground pepper, or to taste
½ cup reserved pasta cooking water

In a large pot of boiling water, cook pasta according to package directions. Drain pasta, reserving 1 cup pasta cooking water. Return pasta to pot. Stir in olive oil, lemon zest, lemon juice, and herbs. Season with salt and pepper. Add some of the reserved pasta cooking water to adjust consistency, if needed.

Serves 7.

(Courtesy: Eden Foods)

We are now departing the land of miraculous parsley. Are you ready to enter a new world of an exotic spice? I'd like you to meet saffron. You may be familiar with it. I assure you that you'll discover some intriguing and fresh benefits of this spice that deserves attention. Plus, it can be used in the Mediterranean diet despite its origin.

HEALING HIGHLIGHTS FROM NATURE'S GARDEN-FEST

✓ Parsley is a good friend herb that is one that deserves to be in your fridge and cupboard for its healing powers.

✓ Like paprika, it is not just a garnish. It is an herb that is super healthy for your immune system.

✓ Research suggests parsley contains cancer-fighting action due to its antioxidants, which may prevent tumors.

✓ Parsley is also packed with vitamins . . . and it is low-cal, low-fat so it's a dieter's friend.

✓ . . . And it gets credit for its diuretic benefits to remedy fluid retention due to pesky hormones like PMS to "peripaws" – when hormones go haywire and women are as nervous as cat.

✓ Parsley is an excellent herb for detoxifying the body, which is an excellent thing to do after overindulging or before a new season.

THE HEALING POWERS OF HERBS AND SPICES

It's always an exciting time
to start your amazing adventures with
herbs and spices.
This photo selection was inspired
by memorable holidays and
four seasons—for you and yours.

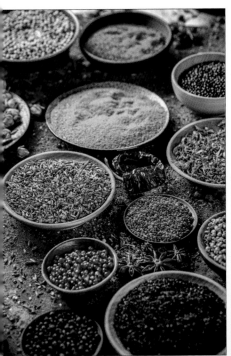

Embrace a new sensory
and savory way of life!
Use herbs and spices
to enhance your dishes
and step up your healthy habits.
*(grafvision/shutterstock.com;
lenetstan/shutterstock.com;
soeka/shutterstock.com)*

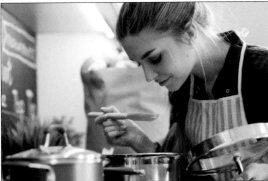

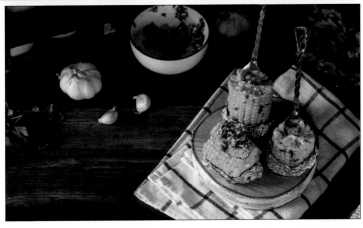

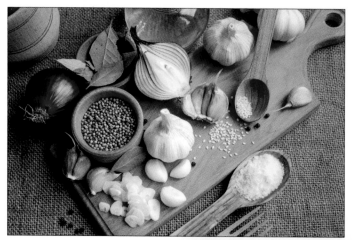

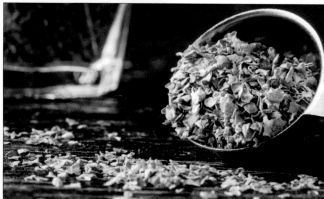

Garlic, a bulb, and marjoram, a leafy herb can really add to the flavor of a dish *(Volodymyr Plysiuk/shutterstock.com; Michelle Lee Photography/shutterstock.com)*

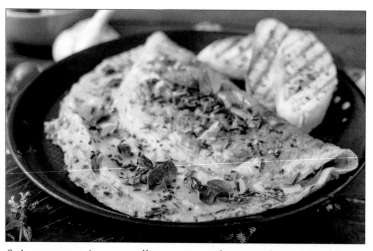

Spicy oregano is an excellent source of antioxidants—and taste! *(Stepanek Photography/shutterstock.com)*

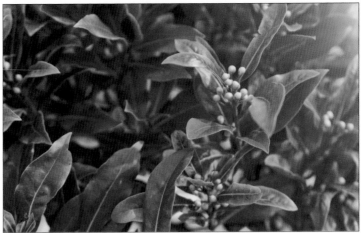

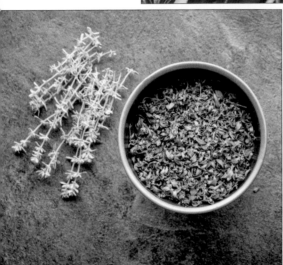

Pairing seasonings will not only improve flavor but also offer a double whammy of good-for-you healing compounds. Bay leaf and thyme are one such magical pairing. *(mrnok/shutterstock.com; Jana Kollarova/shutterstock.com)*

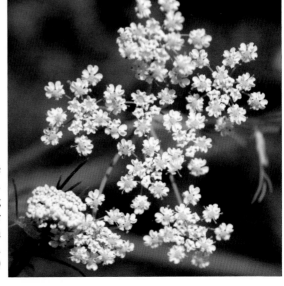

Caraway is a timeless treasure once used by the ancient Greeks. Mediterranean chefs have long understood how much flavor and enjoyment can come from an addition of such herbs and spices. *(Manfred Ruckszio/shutterstock.com)*

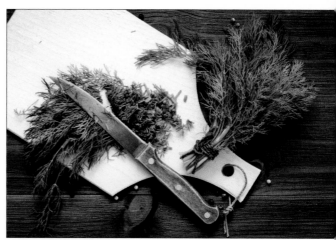

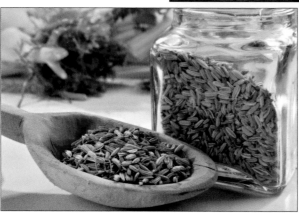

Both dill and fennel are excellent mood enhancers. Feeling a bout of the blues? Add these treats to a dish and get that zap of positivity you need. *(Rui Elena/shutterstock.com; barbajones/shutterstock.com; Elzbieta Sekowska/shutterstock.com)*

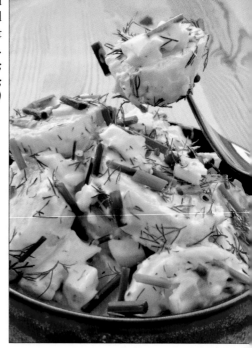

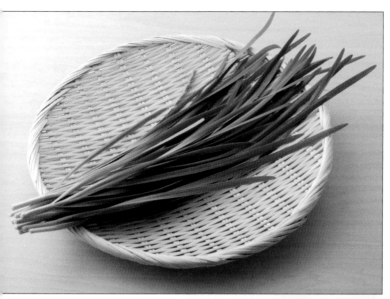

Chives will add aroma and taste—as well as heart-healthy antioxidants—to a wide variety of dishes! (K321/shutterstock.com)

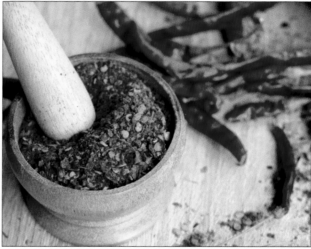

Cayenne has been used to solve plenty of health woes. Seasonal allergies? Use cayenne to combat congestion. Slow metabolism? Add cayenne to your diet to rev it up. (Thanthima Lim/shutterstock.com)

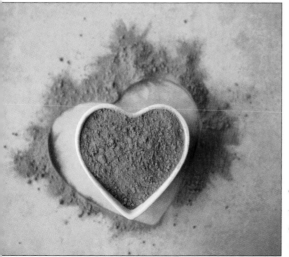

Turmeric is an Indian spice that can be used in a variety of beauty regimens. (Charlotte Lake/shutterstock.com)

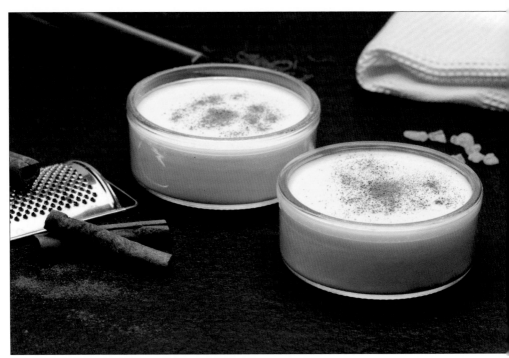

Saffron is a powerful player—it only takes one or two delicate red saffron threads to flavor a dish. Pair it with nutmeg and cinnamon for a beautiful medley of spices. *(Apostolos Mastoris/shutterstock.com)*

Tarragon, an herb often used in French cuisine, can aid in weight loss. Maybe that's how the French stay so thin. *(Kridsada Krongmuang/shutterstock.com)*

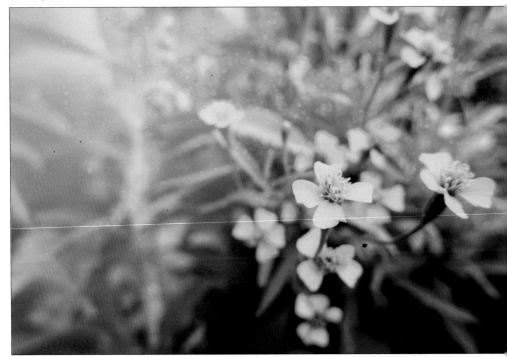

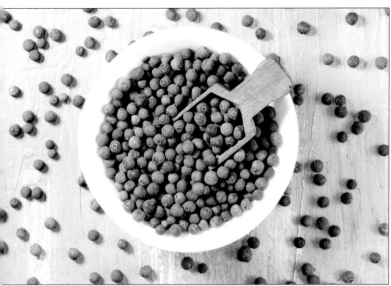

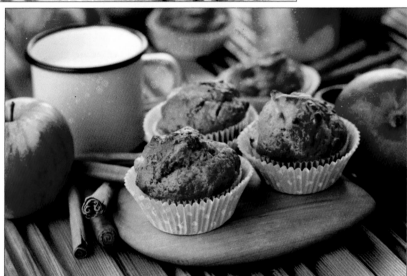

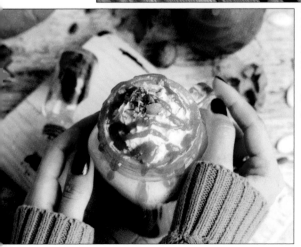

Fall into autumn with allspice! This delicious spice can be used in fun treats, such as apple muffins and pumpkin spice latte. *(zah108/shutterstock.com; matka_Wariatka/shutterstock.com; soeka/shutterstock.com)*

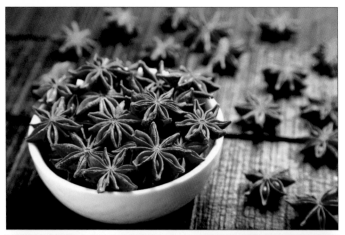

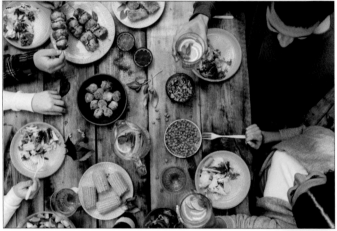

Roll into the holidays with flavorful herbs and spices. Use anise to enhance biscotti— your family and friends will love you for it.
(SAM THOMAS A/shutterstock.com; Maslova Valentina/shutterstock.com; G-Stock Studio/shutterstock.com)

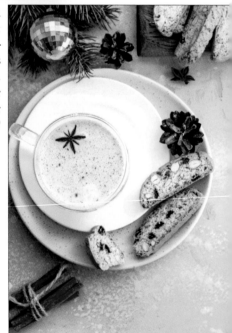

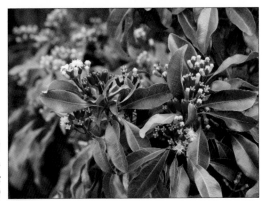

Cooking dinner for a special occasion?
Clove honey glazed ham is sure to delight.
(Denis Moskvinov/shutterstock.com;
K2 PhotoStudio/shutterstock.com)

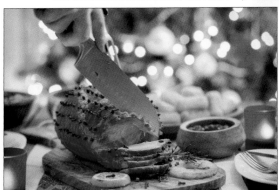

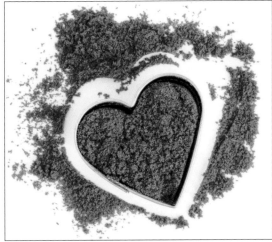

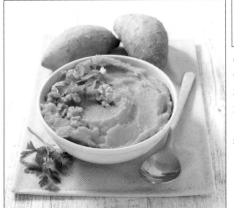

Get ready for another heart-healthy spice
to add an extra something to your side dish.
Smoked paprika will give your sweet potato
mash an extra pizzazz.
(Michelle Lee Photography/shutterstock.com;
margouillat photo/shutterstock.com)

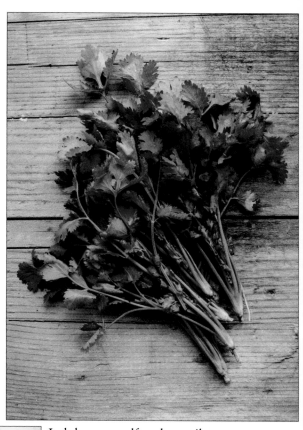

Indulge yourself and use cilantro
for this tasty pull-apart bread.
*(Nelli Syrotynska/shutterstock.com;
Brent Hofacker/shutterstock.com)*

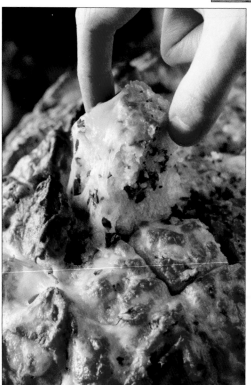

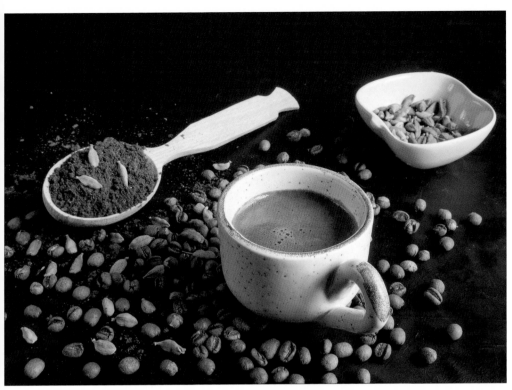

Cardamom is used in both savory and sweet dishes.
This spice can take your banana bread to a whole new level.
(Stanislav71/shutterstock.com; SmileKorn/shutterstock.com)

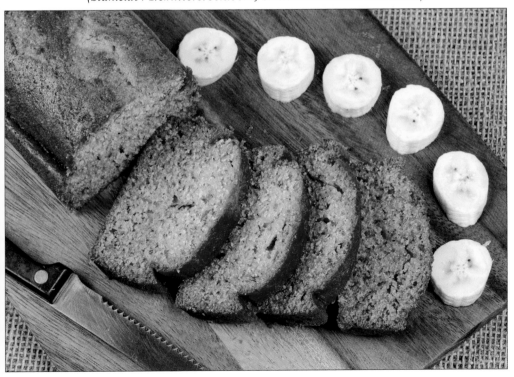

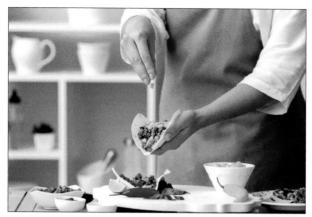

What taco is complete without a kick? Add some cumin to your Mexican dishes for much-needed heat.
(Pixel-Shot/shutterstock.com; SMDSS/shutterstock.com)

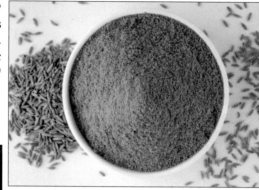

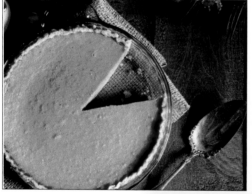

Nutmeg is a warming spice that is sure to make you feel cozy and at home. Use it in your sweet potato pie for an extra treat.
(Lili Blankenhship/shutterstock.com; Puzurin Mihail/shutterstock.com)

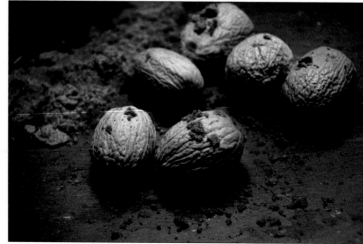

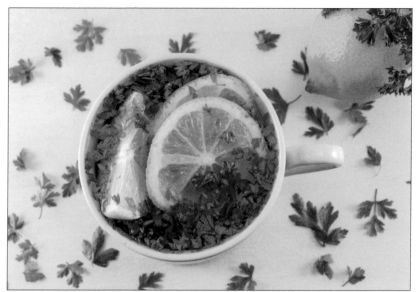

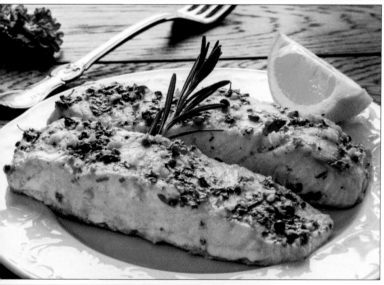

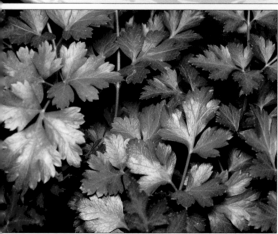

Parsley paired with protein-rich salmon can be a woman's best friend! It's a miracle worker for monthly tummy bloat and weight loss. *(Creative Family/shutterstock.com; Magrig/shutterstock.com; Stephen Orsillo/shutterstock.com)*

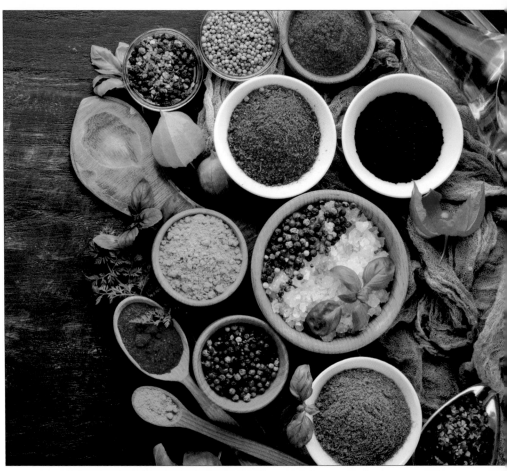

These healing herbs and spices can be used for more than just meals.
Gather together a seasonal medley for some naturally fragrant potpourri.
(YARUNIV Studio/shutterstock.com; fortton/shutterstock.com)

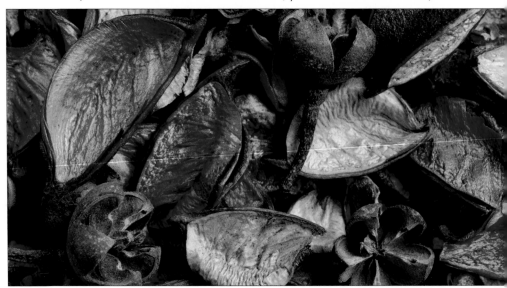

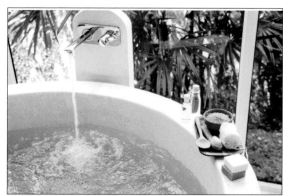

Many luxury spas include herbal treatments in their list of services, such as baths and aromatherapy massages. *(Alena Ozerova/shutterstock.com; MilanMarkovic78/shutterstock.com)*

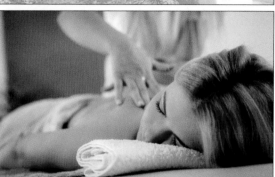

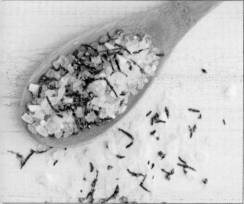

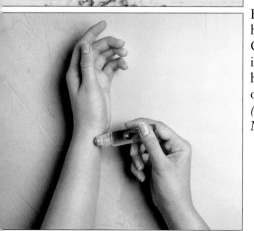

Bring the beauty services home with you. Cardamom is an excellent ingredient to enhance homemade bath salts or perfume rollers. *(Anna Ok/shutterstock.com; New Africa/shutterstock.com)*

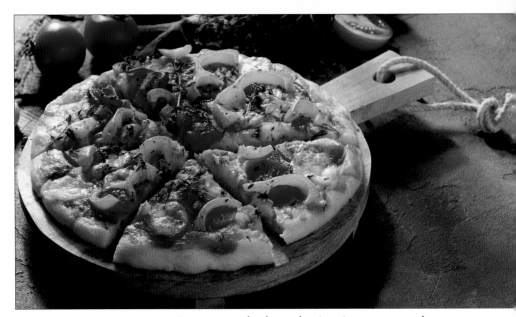

It's so easy to incorporate herbs and spices into your meals, beauty regimens, and lifestyle. Let your imagination take you to new combinations and enjoy the tasty, healthful results. *(Nadezhda Murinets/shutterstock.com; Andrii Horulko/shutterstock.com)*

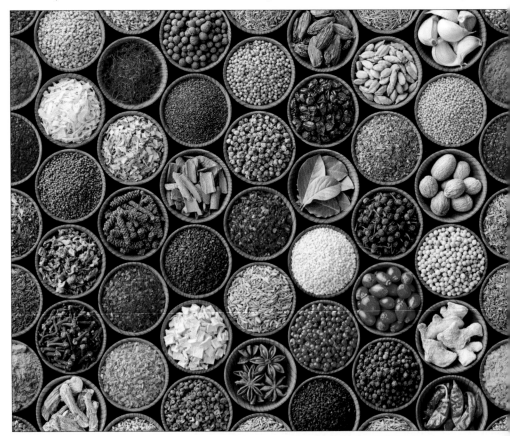

Saffron

(Iridaceae)

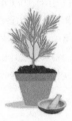

*In saffron-colored mantle from the tides of Oceans
rose the Morning to bright light To gods and men.*
—HOMER, *The Illiad, Book XIX*

One day after a train ride to Quebec City I entered a French shop. It had a chalkboard listing its exotic ice cream flavors. I ordered a cup of saffron gelato. It was yellow, garnished with pistachios on top. The cold treat with a spice from India took me back in time... After my mom returned home from France, she served us spumoni, a dessert: a mix of cherry, chocolate, and pistachio ice creams, layered, in an oval shape and put on a white doily. To make it more special for Christmas Eve, she sprinkled these treats with pistachio nuts and red saffron threads. I pushed the saffron off the ice cream because the fragile strands looked strange like fragile octopi's legs. But as an adult, I discovered the history behind the valuable spice—and I appreciate the delicate treasure.

THE FAMILY TREE OF SAFFRON

No, saffron didn't originally come from Mediterranean countries. Its roots are from Asia. These days, though, it is produced in Spain as well as India, Mexico, and Iran. Herbalists will tell you genuine saffron is pricey, a valuable spice.

It goes back to the seventh century. During that time, it was used in body hygiene and put to work for its medicinal benefits. Herbal historians will tell you ancient Romans used saffron to their baths. Cleopatra, for one, is believed to have soaked in a saffron-infused tub to give her fragrance and glow before a passionate encounter.

SAFFRON PLANT POWER: SURPRISE STUFF

Saffron, not unlike countless herbs, contains carotenoids, which can help enhance everything from eye health to skin disorders. The compounds include picrocrocin and safranal. It is the crocin that provides saffron its golden hue. Saffron also contains anti-inflammatory compounds. Not to forget it contains alpha-carotene, beta-carotene, and zeaxanthin—healing antioxidants.

If you do research, like I did, you will not find an abundance of essential vitamins and nutrients in this spice. It does contain some vitamin A, calcium, folic acid, iron, manganese, magnesium, selenium, riboflavin, and zinc.

More importantly, though, weight-conscious folks will like saffron because it only contains 2 calories in 1 teaspoon. It is low in both sodium and fat. No, it's not a nutrient-dense spice but its antioxidants make it a superspice. Dishes like saffron fregola (an Italian pasta or couscous) served with lamb chops (I saw this item on the dinner menu I scanned when in Toronto, Ontario) are healthy and saffron works with fish and garlic, Mediterranean diet foods.

GROUNDBREAKING DISCOVERIES

Drum roll. Forget the small amounts of nutrients, because the important thing is saffron can help enhance heart health. Research has shown in lab studies that the yellow spice may help lower LDL (bad) cholesterol and lower high blood pressure. And yes, its credit goes to its antioxidant compounds that help lessen plaque from clogging arteries. What's more, it's an anti-inflammatory spice that may also be helpful in lowering your risk of developing heart disease.

Another big plus you'll find in this little spice that is not an underling is that it can help fight depression. Saffron is rich in carotenoids and contains vitamin B (both of these boost the feel-good serotonin chemical found in the body, which plummets due to hormones and even lack of sunshine). Adding saffron in food (15 milligrams of dried saffron twice a day) is advised.

Safety Sound Bite: Avoid if pregnant. Also, small amounts are recommended. Consult with your health practitioner before you try it.

Bountiful Benefits: This herb provides a plethora of healing powers. Herbalists claim it may help guard against arthritis, asthma, depression, pre-menstrual pain (I wish I knew this during my PMS days and nights), and even insomnia.

Also, saffron is touted for its compound crocin, which has an aphrodisiac effect and may enhance touch to be more sensitive and receptive, which can improve lovemaking. It also is a calming substance that is helpful before sex since it lessens performance anxiety. Saffron also has been shown to enhance blood flow—a good thing for men who are having difficulty performing.[1]

Sexy saffron also contains antibacterial properties that can help aid in coughs and even bronchitis. If you've ever suffered from bronchitis, you know too well how the deep cough hurts each time you hack. If saffron is offered in a savory dish or custard, give it a try. Or add it to a cup of tea.

Shake It Up Now! It only takes one or two delicate red saffron threads to flavor a dish. Saffron can be used in appetizers, entrées, desserts, and even beverages. Saffron also comes in the form of yellow powder. I have both forms in my spice cabinet. You can find this spice available at a reasonable price at grocery stores and online. It is said that real saffron is crazy expensive.

Immune Enhancing

Garlic Scallops with Saffron

One holiday season I wanted to cook a memorable meal that would take me back to when I was kid on Christmas Eve. My mom usually made creamed crab over patty shells, but one year she put scallops on the table. So, I followed her lead. I made garlicky scallops with saffron. Dessert? It was a spicy saffron custard. Two types of saffron made two yummy dishes, inspired by my childhood, a place of comfort of good food, herbs, and spices.

¼ *cup fresh lemon juice*
½ *teaspoon saffron*
2 cloves garlic, minced
16 ounces bay scallops
2 cups cooked linguine
Ground pepper to taste
Garnish with fresh parsley

In a nonstick skillet over medium heat, heat the lemon juice, saffron, and garlic. Let simmer. Add the scallops. Sauté until the scallops are opaque, about 3 minutes. Transfer to a bowl. Set aside. In a pan, cover the linguine with water. Follow cooking directions for the pasta. Line a plate with the cooked pasta. Place scallops on the dish. Add ground pepper to taste. Garnish with parsley.

Serves 4.

Saffron Baked Custard

This warm, creamy custard with a spicy kick is easier to bake than taking the gelato route. You don't have to transfer the ingredients to an ice cream maker. Basic egg custard has a history like saffron ice cream. Its roots go back to the Middle Ages. Adding a dash of cardamom provides an India Basundi custard flair to it with almonds, and a few saffron threads with thyme bring it full circle to the Mediterranean region.

2½ cups organic half-and-half
¼ cup granulated white sugar
4 large egg yolks, beaten, room temperature
½ teaspoon cardamom
¼ teaspoon saffron, Spanish threads, chopped (The Spice House)
1 teaspoon nutmeg, ground (The Spice House)
Fresh thyme sprigs and nuts for garnish

Preheat the oven to 350 degrees F. In a bowl combine half-and-half. Add sugar, add egg yolks slowly into half-and-half, stir well. Stir in cardamom and saffron. Pour custard mixture into ramekins. Sprinkle tops with nutmeg. Place into baking dish, add halfway with water. Bake for about 30 minutes or until custard is firm to touch. Do not over bake. Serve warm or cold. Garnish with saffron and thyme.

Serves 4.

Out of the spice cabinet and back to European region to meet and greet another ancient herb. As a healing plant and culinary delight, I predict you are going to fall in love with this extraordinary Mediterranean pick. Give a hand to tarragon, a wonder that deserves its own book.

Healing Highlights from Nature's Garden-Fest

✓ Saffron is an Indian spice but that doesn't mean it didn't make its way to Spain. It is also used to flavor foods in the Mediterranean diet, such as fish and eggs.

✓ True, this spice isn't chock-full of nutrients worthy of a nutrition chart but hold on—neither is honey! But both are rich in protective antioxidants . . .

✓ . . . And medical researchers know saffron acts as an anti-inflammatory, anti-viral, and antibacterial spice that can keep you healthy.

✓ Saffron tea is popular to help guard against respiratory ailments, like colds, flu, and coughs.

✓ This golden spice is known as an exotic and pricey seasoning; the upside more is less, so you can reap its rewards.

✓ Swerve. Saffron can temporarily stain your hands or teeth, like red wine and tea. But note, there are ways like using safe but natural abrasive DIY baking soda and water paste to remedy this issue.

Tarragon

(Asteraceae)

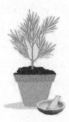

Bait the hook well. This fish will bite.
—WILLIAM SHAKESPEARE

On an autumn weekend my mom served fish with tarragon for dinner.
A French sauce covered the fish in a baking dish. She called it a "deli-
cacy." I stared at my intact trout. "What is this weird stuff?" I asked,
picking at the béarnaise sauce, which savvy chefs create. "Egg yolk, a
shallot, butter, and tarragon leaves," she answered. "Try it, you may
like it." I rebelled hearing the words, "Picky, picky." My mom caved.
She plopped frozen fish sticks from a box on a pan and popped the
kid-friendly fish in the oven . . . Fast-forward to the twenty-first century. Bring on tarragon with its anise flavor for vegetables but hold
the intact fish. Frankly, I wouldn't be able to face my aquarium fish
friends.

THE FAMILY TREE OF TARRAGON

Here comes tarragon, which is called the "dragon herb." The word "tarragon" has a French connection (*herb au dragon,* which is linked to the snake-like shape of the herb's roots). Some herb historians claim its origin may be from Siberia, Russia, and Mongolia, Eastern Asia. As the Herb Society of America tells it, tarragon may have been the weapon to chase away dragons in the Middle Ages.

It grows in Europe, the central and southern regions. The plant has long branches with green leaves and daisy-like flowers (tarragon is in the sunflower family). It is believed to have made its debut in Europe several centuries ago, perhaps around the tenth century when it was brought to Italy. Tarragon was put to use in the past for aiding arthritis, digestion, insomnia, to seasoning food. And its compounds, especially one, make it a multipurpose herb.

TARRAGON PLANT POWER: SURPRISE STUFF

There are two varieties: Russian and French, which is more fragrant. Tarragon, like allspice and cloves, contains eugenol, the pain-relieving compound that is used to soothe gum and toothache pain. This French herb also contains carotenoids (an antioxidant), and phytonutrients.

Tarragon contains some vitamin A, calcium, magnesium, manganese, phosphorus, and potassium. Perhaps its nutrient value is more important as a low-calorie and low-carb spice. One tablespoon of dried tarragon is only 5 calories. Though tarragon isn't a nutrient powerhouse, it is an herb for what it can do for the body.

GROUNDBREAKING DISCOVERIES

Tarragon may help you keep your weight in check; this alone can aid in lowering your odds of heart disease and cancer. But it may also lower blood sugar by improving insulin sensitivity. Lab research has been done, but more studies are needed to prove tarragon can help you maintain blood sugar levels.

Type 2 diabetes is a health problem that affects countless people, both men and women. A middle-aged friend of mine, who worked as a medical assistant in a busy office, was overweight and sedentary. She had signs of diabetes for a while, feeling fatigue to thirsty like a camel. The end result: a visit to the E.R. Her blood sugar levels skyrocketed. Oral meds, diet, and lifestyle changes were doctor's orders. No insulin injections advised. If she could go back in time, she told me she would have given tarragon, like other herbs, a chance, which may have staved off the medical drama.

Bountiful Benefits: Tarragon provides umpteen remedies for health ailments. Due to its array of healing compounds, it can help fight depression, aid in digestion, lessen menstrual cramps, and even beat insomnia. Research shows tarragon is derived from the *Artemisia* group of plants, which may have a relaxing effect and that can help you get adequate sleep—essential to rejuvenate your body. Past studies suggest tarragon contains antibacterial benefits from the essential oil, which can be used as a preservative in foods like cheese. This, in result, can guard against food bacteria.

Shake It Up Now! Tarragon found its way back into my life in vinegar, chocolate truffles, and honey. The French herb has a basil-like flavor and is used in cooking. It is available in dried and packaged fresh leaves at the grocery store and online.

Diet-Friendly

Mediterranean Tarragon Fishcakes with Spinach

Judy Ridgway, food author and judge from the United Kingdom, shares her experience and a spicy fish recipe. "My friends in Spain always use hake for these delicious crisply fishcakes, but you can use any kind of white fish. The best way to cook the fish is to poach it for a very short time in a little milk. Remove the fish from the liquid as soon as the fish turns opaque and you can flake it off the skin or bones. Cook the potatoes in their skins and peel when they are tender.

Tarragon Fishcakes

2 pounds hake, cooked and flaked
1 pound mashed potatoes
1 bunch of spring onions, trimmed and finely chopped
4 tablespoons freshly chopped tarragon
Salt and freshly ground pepper to taste
4 tablespoon sesame seeds
¼ cup fine breadcrumbs
Extra virgin olive oil

Lemon Creamed Spinach

¼ cup heavy cream
8 cups raw spinach, washed and drained
Grated zest of 1 small lemon
Salt and freshly ground black pepper to taste

Carefully mix the fish, potatoes, onions, tarragon, and seasonings, taking care not to break up the flakes of fish too much. Shape into four large cakes and coat with mixed sesame seeds and breadcrumbs. Fry in a hot pan in olive oil for about 5 minutes on each side until the fish cakes are browned and crispy. Meanwhile, heat the cream in a saucepan and gently cook the spinach until it just begins to wilt. Stir in the lemon zest and seasonings. Arrange the cooked spinach on four serving plates and place four cooked fishcakes on top of each serving.

Serves 4 to 8.

(Courtesy: Judy Ridgway)

Another delightful herb is one I enjoy discussing and using. After reading about the merits of thyme I sense you'll feel the same way.

HEALING HIGHLIGHTS FROM NATURE'S GARDEN-FEST

✓ Tarragon, a popular European herb, especially in French cuisine, contains a lot of healthy uses for your body.

✓ Low-cal, low-fat tarragon may help you keep your weight in check, so flavor up fish and vegetables! Weight loss can aid in lowering your odds of heart disease and cancer.

✓ But tarragon is not just a weight-loss herb. Its awesome versatility can help you keep blood sugar levels on keel.

✓ Tarragon has many properties that make magic fighting chronic health ailments, such as depression, insomnia, and pain thanks to its eugenol.

✓ Not only does tarragon aid in healing powers, it is a super culinary herb with flavor to enhance foods in a Mediterranean diet.

Thyme

(Iamiaceae)

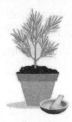

*Those herbs which perfume the air most delightfully,
not passed as the rest, but, being trodden upon and
crushed, are three; that is, burnet, wild thyme and
watermints. Therefore, you are to set whole alleys of
them, to have the pleasure when you walk or tread.*

—FRANCIS BACON

During one Thanksgiving I tried a high-protein diet while house-sitting
for a neighbor. I bought a small turkey. There wasn't a cookbook, culinary utensils, or fresh herbs. I made do with salt and pepper and
popped the under-seasoned poultry into the oven. Hours later, something was missing. No appetizing aroma. The sad turkey was bland. I
tossed it in the trash. But I was hungry. Looking in the freezer, I scored
a bag of cauliflower florets. In a cupboard I discovered store-bought

bottles of dried herbs—including thyme. I boiled the florets and seasoned them with parsley, sage, and thyme. The cauliflower with the
DIY thyme blend was aromatic in contrast to the bird that flopped.
That was the night I dumped a protein diet and turned a new leaf
(pun intended). I vowed to eat more vegetables paired with herbs and
spices—I lost unwanted pounds effortlessly.

THE FAMILY TREE OF THYME

Thyme, a popular, earthy herb, is derived from Southern Europe,
but it is grown throughout Mediterranean countries and Africa to
North America. It is a scented bush that has green leaves and flowers
that can be light pink or purple. Thyme can be traced back to ancient
Egypt for embalming the dead. Ancient Greeks used thyme for its
aroma, whereas Romans used the fragrant herb to cleanse their living
quarters. During ancient Roman times, thyme was believed to protect
people from food poisoning.

In the Middle Ages, the Four Thieves Formula (which not only included cloves as mentioned earlier but other herbs like thyme) is what
robbers used to guard themselves from contracting the deadly bubonic
plague. Thyme, a mighty antiseptic herb, was also believed to provide
courage and stamina in the ancient Roman era. Historians claim Roman
warriors gifted each other with thyme as a symbol of respect and a
badge of courage.

Today, thyme is used to sweeten linens in Europe or even to stuff
pillows, notes the HSA. Also, like me, you probably know thyme is enjoyed as a versatile and delicious culinary herb and garnish in the past
and present.

The Legend of Magical Fairies and Wild Thyme

During the Victorian era, people believed in magical fairies.
Some folks, according to the legend, believed thyme
growing in the woods was a symbol that fairies had been
there. Young girls would go to the forest where wild thyme
grew. The lasses with dreams of good luck, romance, and
prosperity would wait, eagerly wishing to see dancing
good fairies so they could fulfill their desires.

THYME PLANT POWER: SURPRISE STUFF

Earthy thyme may include approximately three hundred different species, points out the Herb Society of America. The herb contains antioxidants, including apigenin, lutein, zeaxanthin, and thymol—the primary antiseptic compound that gives the herb its distinct flavor. This Mediterranean herb contains a high antioxidant rating, like cloves and chives, on the ORAC scale.

Thyme also boasts plenty of healthy vitamins and minerals. The lineup includes vitamin A, vitamin C, and vitamin E. Also, thyme contains B-complex vitamins and folic acid. The minerals are to be noted, too, such as iron, magnesium, manganese, potassium, and selenium.

THYME NUTRIENTS

Here are some basic nutrients found in 100 grams or ½ cup of fresh thyme, according to the USDA National Nutrient Database.

Calories	101
Calcium	405 milligrams
Dietary fiber	14 grams
Iron	17.45 milligrams
Magnesium	160 milligrams
Phosphorus	106 milligrams
Potassium	609 milligrams
Protein	5.56 grams
Sodium	9 milligrams

GROUNDBREAKING DISCOVERIES

It is not surprising that thyme is a heart-healthy herb, which is of interest because heart disease is still the number one cause of death. Give credit to thyme's minerals such as potassium. Potassium can lessen the stress on the cardiovascular system. How? Simply put, the mineral, also found in fruits and vegetables, relaxes blood vessels and lowers blood pressure. Over time, keeping your blood pressure numbers normal at 120 over 80 (or even a bit under) may help to lessen the risk of developing heart attacks and strokes.

Not to forget the immunity-boosting vitamin C is in this herb. We know vitamin C can boost white blood cells, which are the good guys that strengthen the body's immune system. A weakened immune response can make us more vulnerable to contracting a common cold, flu bug, or even cancer. Potential medicinal powers of phytochemicals and medicinal herbs, like thyme, used for cancer prevention are not a pipe dream. Research shows thyme contains terpenoids, reported in studies for their cancer preventive properties. Other anti-cancer compounds in thyme include borneol, carvacoel, geraniol, sabine hydrate, and thymol.[1]

Bountiful Benefits: Thyme is touted for its multiple advantages. Past research shows that thyme has anti-inflammatory compounds. That fact makes thyme a useful herb for aiding respiratory ailments, including bronchitis, seasonal allergies, colds, and coughs. Since it works as an anti-inflammatory, it may open up your airways and can help you breathe easier.

It is also believed to stimulate blood circulation, thanks to its iron content of almost 20 percent of the recommended daily value. Iron stimulates red blood cells, enhancing circulation and oxygen to organs in the body. As a teenager I was borderline anemic due to crash diets from peer pressure to be thin. In my golden years, when I get a checkup my oxygen levels are monitored. Living in the mountains with high altitude doesn't help, but a healthy lifestyle can counteract getting adequate oxygen. Thyme is a good source of iron that both women and men should include in their diet.

Thyme also staves off fungal infections, and even relieves stress (raise your hand if you need help in this area), which can lead to chronic health issues such as elevated blood pressure or lower immunity to colds and flu. The vitamin C in thyme boosts white blood cells, which are like an army of soldiers protecting the body's immune system. Plus, vitamin C helps produce collagen, needed to repair blood vessels, cells, muscles, and tissues.

This herb can also help guard against respiratory ailments like pesky seasonal allergies that come with a mixed bag of itchy eyes and throat, sneezing, and headaches. (The spring and autumn pollen and ragweed in the mountains are not my friends.) I did befriend thyme and added it to my arsenal to fight allergens.

During one winter when people on social media complained of a flu bug and colds, I (the hypochondriac) made a rustic shepherd's meatless pie baked with fresh thyme. The distinct herb taste is a flavorful peppery oregano flavor.

Safety Sound Bite: Do not overindulge in thyme because it may cause gastrointestinal discomfort.

Shake It Up Now! Thyme can be put to use both fresh and dried. I like combining both types for flavor and texture in lemon cookies and scones. It is an ingredient used in hand sanitizers, mouthwash, and even some toothpastes. Thyme is often used dried and used in wreaths past and present-day. When tracking Dr. Will Clower's sailing around the world, stopping in Las Palmas, a city in the Canary Islands, thyme was noted. He spoke of thyme sauce with fish for dinner. I cooked up salmon from the butcher and added thyme sprigs plucked from my potted plant as I studied herbs and spices on the deck of my Tahoe cabin.

The leaves can be removed from the stems and ground into spice, or the sprigs can be added in cooking. Leaves and sprigs can be used in tea and in homemade household cleaning products and crafts. It is available in both fresh (I buy the organic variety in a container; a pot to grow in my kitchen in the summer) and dried form at the grocery store. Also, thyme is used in spice blends, such as herbes de Provence and zaatar.

Immune-Boosting

Roasted Cauliflower with Thyme

In my childhood, my mother served cauliflower topped with a cheddar cheese sauce. Instead of using high fat cheese to make vegetables tasty, thyme paired with garlic and spices can titillate the palate. This is an easy dish that can be served year-round, but is perfect to warm you up during autumn and winter. Also, you can make a comforting cauliflower soup or cauliflower steaks. (Slice a whole cauliflower in thick slices and proceed as you will with florets.) This herby recipe is not mine but I treat it like it is.

1 medium cauliflower cut into florets
1 large red onion, sliced into 1-inch-thick wedges
4 tablespoons Eden Extra Virgin Olive Oil
4 cloves garlic, unpeeled
4 sprigs fresh thyme
4 teaspoon Eden Sea Salt
¼ teaspoon garlic salt, or to taste
⅛ teaspoon black pepper, or to taste

Preheat the oven to 425 degrees F. Place all ingredients in a medium mixing bowl and toss to evenly coat the cauliflower and onions with oil and seasonings. Transfer to a large rimmed baking sheet and bake for 50 to 60 minutes or until tender and browned, tossing occasionally to evenly roast. Remove and place in a serving dish.

Serves 4.

(Courtesy: Eden Foods)

Now I'm ready to talk turmeric. I admit I learned a lot of intriguing facts when doing my turmeric research. Are you ready to find out what I discovered? Read on.

Healing Highlights from Nature's Garden-Fest

✓ Thyme is a popular Mediterranean herb from ancient days in Europe. It was one of the herbs used in the antibacterial Four Thieves Formula to protect against the deadly plague.

✓ Thymol is the compound in thyme responsible for its aroma and healing powers such as antiseptic qualities to fight germs and bacteria . . .

✓ The antimicrobial compounds help guard the body against infections and enhances the immune system—important for people of all ages.

✓ Thyme also contains minerals, such as potassium, helpful to keep blood pressure healthy and keep heart disease at bay.

✓ This herb when used fresh is pretty as a garnish for soups, stews, breads, and cakes. Fresh sprigs are attractive, but combining both dried and fresh crumbled leaves also adds texture and flavor . . .

✓ Thyme can be cooked for a long time and still retain its healing compounds for your health's sake.

Turmeric

(Zingiberacea)

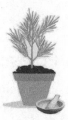

That Spices fly In the Receipt—
It was the Distance—Was Savory . . .
—EMILY DICKENSON, *Undue Significance a starving man*
attaches

As a thirty-something journalist living in the San Francisco Bay Area, I was invited to dinner by my neighbor, an adventurous architect-foodie who took a fancy to foreign cuisine. At a rustic Indian shop around the corner from my bungalow, I felt on edge. Memories of my worldly mom's yellow curried rice dishes started to haunt me. I ordered a veggie burger spiked with turmeric. But that spicy turmeric burger was edible. I give credit to the chef, my date, and turmeric, which is edible if it is used sparingly. That day was another reminder to me to be more adventurous in trying new flavors—like new things—for the thrill of living life in the moment and to its fullest.

THE FAMILY TREE OF TURMERIC

Turmeric, also called Indian saffron, comes from the Curcuma long plant. It originated in Southeast India and Asia and has been used for centuries. It is best known for ancient use as a dye and in folk medicine for a variety of health ailments.

The Herbal Society of America confirms herbalists' observations about turmeric's roots (literally). The turmeric plant is a tropical one and it grows about three feet tall. The underground stem of the plant grows into a bulbous shape, much like fresh ginger (it is also related to the ginger family). It is the root that is boiled, dried, and then crushed into powder.

TURMERIC PLANT POWER: SURPRISE STUFF

The Indian superspice is super thanks to its mighty compound curcumin and related compounds known as curcuminoids—the chemicals that give this spice its healing powers. Turmeric contains antioxidant vitamins C and E.

One tablespoon of turmeric is only approximately 23 calories. It also contains some minerals and vitamins, some significant to meet percentages of your daily value needs: manganese, 26 percent; iron, 16 percent; and vitamin B6, magnesium, potassium, and 1.4 grams of dietary fiber.

GROUNDBREAKING DISCOVERIES

Past research has shown it may be that curcuminoids found in turmeric can help lessen inflammation in diseases and health ailments. Many herbs and spices, like turmeric, offer anti-inflammatory compounds that have healing powers, since inflammation is a culprit in ailments such as arthritis and diseases—even cancer.[1]

Research shows turmeric has antifungal and antibacterial compounds, which may be helpful in staving off viruses that affect the immune system. Cancer, which is linked to the immune response, may be bolstered by the spice. The National Center for Complementary and Integrative Health has studied turmeric and its curcumin.

Scientists say it may be helpful for treatment of prostate and colon cancer. There are a lot of lab studies that show turmeric can help tumors from forming or stop cancer cells from spreading. Not to forget the American Institute for Cancer Research has noted turmeric, like garlic, may help to guard against cancer.

Turmeric may also play a role in heart health, lessening plaque buildup in the arteries. That means turmeric can help unclog arteries, which can lower the risk of developing heart attacks and strokes. Of course, this spice isn't a magic cure-all pill guaranteed to work miracles. But including it in a heart-healthy Mediterranean diet couldn't hurt, especially when it has so many additional advantages.

Bountiful Benefits: Thanks to its curcumin contents, turmeric is believed to tweak brain chemicals and may lessen depression in the same way as antidepressant meds like fluoxetine. It is believed to aid in digestion, enhance mental alertness, improve blood sugar levels, and even provide pain relief due to its anti-inflammatory compounds by usage of a poultice. But note, the yellowish color of turmeric can stain when used topically. Using a paste of baking soda and water can eliminate the color on your hands or teeth.

Safety Sound Bite: Turmeric may interfere with blood-thinning and diabetes medications. Do not used if pregnant. Before adding this spice to your diet, consult with your health practitioner.

Shake It Up Now! Turmeric is used mainly in Indian and Thai dishes. Healthful legumes, poultry, rice, and yogurt include turmeric and are all part of the Mediterranean diet. Turmeric is used for a variety of things, including butters, curry powders, mustards, ice cream, and to color foods and cosmetics. It is available in powder and found easily at grocery stores and online. Also, turmeric supplements and a wide variety of tea combinations are available online and at health food stores.

Anti-Inflammatory

Mediterranean Salad with Turmeric Dressing

Turmeric is a popular spice known for its intense flavor that adds a kick to vegetables sometimes needing seasoning. Since I'm not a true fan of Indian cuisine (which includes foods like tandoori chicken or fish and yogurt cucumber salad), pairing turmeric with Mediterranean fare works for me. Putting turmeric in a dressing with olive oil, and herbs and spices from European countries, is a smart way to get health benefits of the exotic spice. This recipe is inspired by the Indian dinner date but repurposed to my personal preference for Mediterranean food.

½ cup baby spinach
½ cup kale
1 Roma tomato, chopped
1 teaspoon red onion, chopped
¼ cup feta cheese, crumbled
⅛ cup cranberries, dried
2 teaspoons walnuts, chopped

TURMERIC DRESSING

1 tablespoon extra virgin olive oil
1 tablespoon fresh lemon juice
½ teaspoon turmeric powder
¼ teaspoon fresh thyme
¼ teaspoon fresh parsley
¼ teaspoon black pepper
2 tablespoons Parmesan shavings

In a small bowl, whisk oil, juice, turmeric, thyme, parsley, and pepper. Place greens, tomato, onion, cheese, berries, and nuts on a salad plate. Drizzle with dressing. Sprinkle with cheese.

Serves 1.

In my new, improved herb and spice cabinet, we've come to the end of the 22 picks. This selection of seasonings with a Mediterranean twist does not imply that's all there is in the world of herbs and spices. In the next chapter, you're going to be treated to a mixed bag of spice blends used for cooking and baking. Some blends you may be familiar with and are in your kitchen cupboard. Others will be an exciting novelty for you as they were to me. Come along now, as the spicy adventure continues . . .

HEALING HIGHLIGHTS FROM NATURE'S GARDEN-FEST

✓ An Indian spice is in a Mediterranean mix of herbs and spices? Um, yes! True, its roots are not European but it did make its way to Spain.

✓ Turmeric has so many health benefits it would be sinful to leave it out of the chosen 22 herbs and spices.

✓ This spice contains anti-inflammatory properties, which make it a powerful healer for guarding against health ailments and diseases.

✓ It is the compound curcumin in turmeric that is pinpointed by researchers and found to be the active ingredient to fight illness.

✓ Do not let the exotic spice sit in the cupboard if you don't prefer it in food! Bring it on for all of its topical uses . . .

✓ . . . If you don't like the taste of turmeric, you may find you love it in flavored teas or use it topically!

✓ Refer to the folk remedies chapter to find out how a paste can help treat health ailments, and it even works in beauty regimens.

The Blends

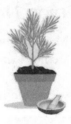

Spice a dish with love and it pleases every palate.
—PLAUTUS

In the summer of 1999, I stocked the pantry with canned and boxed goods. I didn't include dried herbs and spices—the blends. When 2000 arrived—the planet continued to exist—but I was stuck with processed survival foodstuff.

My first snowy night in the Tahoe cabin, I grabbed a few russet potatoes and sliced them into steak fry–size pieces. I put them in a baking dish. I didn't have any fresh herbs and spices. And that was the night I met herbes de Provence—a blend of dried Mediterranean spices.

I drizzled the taters with melted butter. Then, I sprinkled the blend on top. Once the potatoes were golden and crispy, I bit into the first fry. It was love at first bite. Not one but five herbs on my potatoes made my herbes de Provence French fries a culinary delight. I was hooked by the amazing five-in-one flavor blend. Now, whenever I travel away from home, herby fries are a food that warms me up, especially if there are plenty of herbs and spices.

HERE COME THE BRILLIANT BLENDS

The blends—a mishmash of herbs and spices—changes up dishes, like pasta plates to hot sandwiches, soups, and homemade breads. The blends opened up a whole new world to me. I am a devoted fan of herb and spice blends. Sure, fresh herbs are my first choice, but in reality, unless you live on an herb farm you won't always have access to it. If you want to use cilantro for pesto sauce or thyme for biscuits it may not be in season, you forgot to pick it up at the store, or it's too pricey. Enter my much-loved mixes.

Chili Powder (Spicy): Did you know? Chili powder is a blend of many spices, including cayenne, which only is one-seventh of the mix. It is a spicy blend of ancho chile, cumin, Mexican oregano, and paprika. It's good with dry rubs, sauces, and soups. Jessicka Nebesni of the Eugene, Oregon-based Mountain Rose Herbs is a chili powder enthusiast. When I asked her if she was stranded on a deserted island and she could only pick one spice, she assured me chili powder is her choice. Here, see why it's her favorite . . .

The spicy blend can be used internally and also topically, making it very useful in everyday life. Nebesni knows it is "great to have on hand in situations where you could be called on to do more physical activity. Making soothing muscle rubs with this ingredient is one of my favorite uses, though I am a board-spectrum chili enjoyer." It can be a morning tonic with some warm water, apple cider vinegar, and honey, she adds: "Talk about getting a jump start to your day!"

Five-Spice Powder (Sweet): No, this spice blend is not European but it does include fennel seeds, a Mediterranean spice. The mix is of Chinese cinnamon, cloves, fennel seeds, star anise, and Sichuan pepper. Since it is a combination of spices the healing powers are the same but you get a super dose of health benefits since you're using a combination. It complements vegetables and pairs well with garlic, a Mediterranean favorite.

Greek Mediterranean Seasoning (Spicy): There are many variations of a basic European blend. The Spice House makes it simple. Three ingredients are the blend: Greek oregano, garlic, and lemon peel. There are spin-offs, including chiles, bell peppers, and even salt but the trio works nicely.

Herbes de Provence (Earthy): It is a Mediterranean mix of dried herbs (and occasionally spices) used in cuisine from Provence in France. The blend can include oregano, rosemary, sage, tarragon, and thyme. It can also contain fennel seeds, lavender, and savory. It wasn't named herbes de Provence until the seventies in North America, but the herbs were used for centuries.

The Herb Society of America's education coordinator Karen Kennedy says, "I love rosemary because it is both a refreshing herb and one that complements a variety of flavors in food." The herb expert adds, "Rosemary is often associated with memory. Greek scholars wore a garland of rosemary on their heads to help their memory during examinations. I'm fond of the flavor that it imparts. The fact that rosemary is full of antioxidants is a bonus!"

Herbes de Provence contains the same medicinal benefits of the herb, including rosemary, I cover in this book. It is touted for its antibacterial advantages. Best uses: dry rubs, soups, salad dressings. Food pairings: fish, poultry, vegetables (eggplant, potatoes, tomatoes).

Italian Seasoning (Savory): Not unlike herbes de Provence, it is a mix of basil, oregano, rosemary, savory, and thyme. This mix of herbs all have anti-inflammatory, antibacterial health benefits. Use in herb breads, pasta, pizza, and Italian cuisine, including fish and poultry.

I personally use it on a quick pasta dish to provide flavor for a convenient dinner, such as penne pasta with Roma tomatoes, cruciferous vegetables, sprinkled with Italian seasoning and topped with Parm shavings. Fresh herbs are more attractive and can be more flavorful—but this Italian blend does please the palate in a pinch (during a snowstorm or when there isn't time to buy fresh herbs).

You can whip up a DIY Italian blend combining many of my top herbs and spices 22 picks: In a bowl, mix it up with 2 tablespoons cayenne, 2 tablespoons garlic powder, 2 tablespoons marjoram, 2 tablespoons oregano, 2 tablespoons paprika, and 2 tablespoons thyme. Makes about ¾ cup. Put in covered container.

Savory, a Summer and Winter Herb

Savory isn't in my 22 picks but it is found in the blends and is a Mediterranean treasure—and Karen Kennedy of the Herb Society of America dishes on savory. It is one of her favorite seasonal herbs. Read on, to get her personal take on this special chosen one . . .

The original botanical name of most savories is *Satureja*. Many plants that were once in this genus, and which are still commonly called savories, now belong to the genera *Micromeria*, *Clinopodium*, *Calamintha*, and *Acinos*. Savory is known as the "bean herb" (*bohnenkraut* in German) because it both enhances the flavor of beans and also helps in their digestion, thus decreasing the flatulence often associated with these and other legumes. I love the flavor of both winter and summer savory, similar to a combination of oregano and thyme, it adds to soups and stews.

Indeed, savory is used in summer and winter dishes but the dried form is available year-round. The aroma of this herb is similar to marjoram and thyme. Winter savory with dark green leaves is stronger in flavor. Savory is an herb found in some herbes de Provence and Italian seasoning blends. Savory is touted for its antiseptic and digestive medicinal advantages—and French herbalists claim it may help enhance sex drive. But note, summer savory is the sexy herb, whereas winter savory may put a damper on finding that loving feeling. You may have to settle for a gastronomic lovefest when ingesting savory during the chill of Old Man Wintertime. Or perhaps, to feel amorous on a cold night, savor a cayenne-infused chocolate square after eating a bowl of hot savory stew.

Ras El-Hanout (Savory): The Great America Spice Company who shared this spice blend with me knows the history behind this spice mixture. It means "top of the shop." The spice mixture is used in Moroccan cooking and its purpose is to provide and African flavor. It contains more than twenty-five ingredients (many of my Mediterranean picks), including allspice, cardamom, cayenne, chives, cloves, cumin, and turmeric. It is spicy and sweet with its mixture of herbs and spices. It's best used to season casseroles, couscous, and vegetables. It's recommended to add chickpeas for an exciting burst of flavor! I chose to use ras el-hanout in a vegetarian shepherd's pie made with russet potatoes, tomatoes, zucchini, fresh garlic, shallots, and mozzarella cheese. The herb and spice blend gave my signature casserole Mediterranean flavors to this dish—without meat or poultry!

Spicy Meatless Shepherd's Pie

I'm talking fresh vegetables, fresh herbs—and a spice blend. I've made a variety of shepherd pie recipes—but this one is super flavorful. It is a winter savory delight because of the spice blend ras-el-hanout. No frozen taters or canned vegetables are used for this version. The Spicy Meatless Shepherd's Pie is inspired by my past traveling adventures where fresh food, herbs, and spices are not available.

3 large russet potatoes
¼ cup 2 percent organic low-fat milk
2 tablespoons European-style butter
1 teaspoon fresh garlic, minced
2 sprigs thyme and 2 sprigs rosemary, chopped
¼ teaspoon nutmeg
1 teaspoon ras-el-hanout
½ cup lentils, cooked (optional)
1 cup fresh cruciferous vegetables, broccoli, chopped
1 tablespoon each olive oil and unsalted butter
¾ to 1 cup tomatoes, chopped
½ cup Parmesan cheese, grated
½ cup Monterey Jack, shredded
Ground black pepper to taste
Fresh parsley, chopped for garnish

In a large pot, fill with water and place washed potatoes. Boil until tender and rinse under cold water; peel skins. (Or you can nuke them in the microwave and leave skins on.) Put potatoes into a mixing bowl. Add milk and butter. Fold in garlic, thyme, rosemary, nutmeg, and ras-el-hanout. Mash until smooth. Or keep it chunky if preferred for a rustic dish. Set aside. Sauté lentils and crucifer vegetables in olive oil and butter or nuke in a bowl of water until tender and drain. Preheat the oven to 350 degrees F. Place cooked lentils and cruciferous vegetables into a medium-size round baking dish. Spread potato herbal and spice mixture on top of vegetables. Top with tomatoes. Sprinkle cheeses on top. Bake for about 20 to 25 minutes or until cheese bubbles and top is slightly golden. Sprinkle with pepper and parsley.

Serves 4 to 6.

Za'atar: I was reluctant to try this blend because I wasn't familiar with a few of the herbs and spices. Remember, I'm the picky rabbit food eater from California. This Middle East blend uses oregano and thyme as a base, but also a mixture of some of my Mediterranean picks, including cumin, dill, fennel seeds, marjoram, and parsley. Not to forget it contains black pepper, mint, salt, sesame seed, savory, sumac, and orange peel. I followed the Great America Spice company's recommendation: I mixed a dash or two of the blends with 1 teaspoon of extra virgin olive oil. I drizzled it over a hot multigrain bagel fresh from the local bakery. It was a gastronomic explosion of herbal flavors from the first bite to the last. You can mix Za'atar with olive oil or hummus for dips.

Pumpkin Spice Is Hot Stuff (Spicy Recipes)

Ah, pumpkin spice! This blend is full of autumn's warming spices, including cinnamon, cloves, ginger, and nutmeg (and sometimes allspice). This blend goes back to the late 1800s. Big and small spice companies offer it. Personally, I have containers from McCormick and Mountain Rose Herbs; and I've made it myself, too. Pumpkin spice is a blend used in pumpkin pie, bread, scones, and sprinkled on top of a latte. Pumpkin spice is a popular trend and store-bought foods are infused with it during the holiday season. This spice blend is also used for savory dishes, such as a baked squash dish.

Is it health-giving? Since pumpkin spice includes many spices with healing compounds, you're getting more of the good for your properties. I've read articles stating that the pumpkin spice trend is over, but then every year it's ba-a-ck! In fact, some makers are going overboard and adding pumpkin spice in everything, from bagels to pretzels. Here are two of my favorite recipes—fudge and French toast—using pumpkin spice, but the uses of this spice blend are limitless.

Pumpkin Spice Walnut Fudge

Perhaps I love pumpkin spice fudge because it's a sign of autumn. This recipe is inspired by my late "fairy godmother" who knew how to enjoy life's spicy pleasures (she lived to one hundred). She insisted on gifting me one pound of this spicy candy for my birthday . . . ah, the flavors and aroma linger in my mind. No wonder I created this recipe with the notes of pumpkin spice.

¼ cup pumpkin puree
½ cup European-style butter
⅓ cup organic 2 percent low-fat milk
4 cups confectioners sugar
2 teaspoons pumpkin spice (Mount Rose Herbs)
¾ cup walnuts, chopped
1 tablespoon European-style butter

In a bowl, combine pumpkin and butter. Put in microwave a few minutes until it bubbles. Remove. Add milk. Set aside. In a large bowl, sift 4 cups of sugar. Add pumpkin mixture. Stir well. Add spice and walnuts. Grease an 8-inch by 8-inch pan with butter. Put in fudge mixture. Spread evenly. Cover with foil and place into refrigerator for two hours. Remove and place pan on cutting board. You can remove the entire square onto the board. Cut into squares. Place each one into a small cupcake wrapper.

Makes 16 to 20 pieces.

Store in a covered container inside the refrigerator.

Pumpkin Spice French Toast

I experienced pumpkins lining the cobblestone sidewalks in Quebec City, Quebec, while sipping a spiced coffee. A pretty pumpkin patch in the Apple Hill area of Placerville, south of Lake Tahoe, greeted me during Indian summer. I made an apple pie with a spice blend. Instead of a pumpkin pie, scones, or fudge—I have made all three in my rustic cabin in the mountains—warm up to making Pumpkin French Toast with pumpkin spice.

1 teaspoon European-style butter
2 eggs, large, brown
½ cup low-fat organic milk
¼ cup pumpkin puree
1 teaspoon organic pumpkin spice (Mountain Rose Herbs)
½ teaspoon cinnamon

½ teaspoon vanilla extract
4 slices brioche bread (the thicker, the better)
Honey for drizzling
European-style butter, extra for topping
Nuts for garnish (pecans or walnuts, chopped)

In a large frying pan over medium heat, melt butter. Set aside. In a bowl, combine eggs, milk, pumpkin, spices, and vanilla. Mix well. Dunk bread slices (both sides) into the egg mixture. Place each slice into the pan. Medium heat is recommended. Cook for a few minutes and turn over. Repeat until golden brown. Serve hot. Add a pat of butter, drizzle with honey, and sprinkle nuts.

Serves 2.

This recipe is easy to put together. Not only is it quick, it's versatile. It is good for breakfast, especially paired with chunks of seasonal fruit, and a cup of hot pumpkin spice flavored coffee or tea. But it can suffice as a late-night snack, too. The pumpkin touch is fall-ish. The best part: It won't be tricked, like the South Shore pumpkin that came to my cabin and never lived a full life.

MORE BAKING SPICE BLENDS

Apple Pie Spice: A popular blend used in autumn and winter. It is a mixture of allspice, cinnamon, and nutmeg. It can also contain cardamom, cloves, or ginger. Apple pie spice is used in apple pie, cookies, crisps and crumbles, and muffins.

Cinnamon-Sugar: I've tried mixing cinnamon and sugar without measuring and it just isn't a perfect concoction. A store-bought variety is convenient to use. The ratio is 1/2 cup granulated sugar with 1 tablespoon cinnamon. It is commonly used on cinnamon toast to sprinkling on top of oatmeal, homemade muffins, pies, and cookies.

English Mixed Spice: It is an English blend of allspice, cloves, coriander, mace, and nutmeg—and on occasion cinnamon. You can enjoy this traditional mix in a batch of scones, sweet fruit, and nut bread, or muffins paired with tea.

The bottom line: I've shared with you some favorite and flavorful Mediterranean blends. But you'll discover there are a wide variety of other blends that will fit your blend fancy. Blends for cooking and baking are a cook's best friend, whether it's a storm or an impromptu meal happens—you're covered.

Germ Safeguarding

Herbes de Provence Oven-Baked Fries

During springtime I was bound for Toronto, Ontario. It was eerie and exciting to visit a province I hitchhiked to with a dog in my twenties. Then, it happened. At 5:30 A.M. I boarded the aircraft at Reno-Tahoe International Airport. A man was having difficulty fitting his steel carry-on into the compartment; he accidentally slammed my face with the luggage. Despite the blow, I carried on to Canada. Once in the foreign country and inside a foreign hotel room my face was swollen and bruised. Icing on my cheek, I ordered room service: fries: Parm, garlic, chopped herbs, and caper aioli (a golden Mediterranean sauce made of garlic and olive oil). The spicy taters were hot and crispy but soft inside. The combo of herbs and potatoes helped me to chill. I savored the garlic fries while overlooking a panoramic view of the city and Lake Ontario. Perhaps the anti-inflammatory effect of garlic helped a bit; in the morning the swelling had gone down. I survived.

2 large potatoes, rinsed with water (or sweet, russet, New)
¼ cup European-style butter and/or olive oil

A dash of ground pepper, garlic powder, and paprika
2 teaspoons herbes de Provence (Mountain Rose
Herbs)
¼ cup Parmesan cheese (shavings or shredded)
Sea salt (optional)
Parsley (fresh or dried) for garnish
Ketchup (for dipping)

Preheat the oven to 400 degrees F. On a cutting board, slice potatoes with a sharp knife. You can make thick wedges or thin slices like I did. Place on a non-stick cookie sheet. Drizzle with melted butter or oil. Sprinkle tops with pepper, garlic powder, paprika, herbes de Provence, and Parm cheese. Bake for about 15 minutes. Turn fries. Bake another 15 minutes. Turn off oven and let rest for about 20 minutes. Place fries in two bowls. Sprinkle with sea salt and parsley. Drizzle or dip into ketchup.

Makes 2 servings.

Tip: Allowing the potatoes to bake at a hot heat, turning, and leaving in the oven makes them oh-so crispy.

Now that I've brought out my collection of the blends, it's time to put them away. Or not. Herbs and spices can help you age gracefully. Whether you're looking to slim down or up your game to stall the biological aging clock—it's time for seasonings. Time is a wasting, as the country song lyrics goes. Come along, this next age-fighting part is super multi-generational.

We are now entering the land of learning how to use herbs and spices to help enhance the quality and quantity of your lifespan. No kidding.

Healing Highlights from Nature's Garden-Fest

✓ Spice blends are not something to ignore or exclude from your spice rack—not a chance. Once you use one or two, you'll likely wonder, "How did I survive without this blend?"

✓ A spice blend like herbes de Provence is brilliant because you get multiple healing benefits because of the mix of herbs . . .

✓ And the amazing combo of herbs and spices spells convenience. Not to ignore the flavors of blends that give life to bland dishes as well as sauces and soups.

✓ Cooking with the blends provides different flavors to superfoods in the Mediterranean diet . . .

✓ . . . And the baking blends add year-round spice to cookies and pies to cakes and scones, an added edge when it comes to pleasing the palate . . .

✓ Don't forget blends spice up fish to poultry . . . providing that extraordinary wow factor and adventurous taste and texture to each dish.

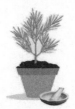

PART 3

AGE-DEFYING HERBS AND SPICES

Season Up, Slim Down

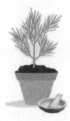

Fear is the spice that makes it interesting to go ahead.
—Daniel Boone

One fall day during a doctor's check-up after booking a long-anticipated trip to Alaska, I asked the question. "Should I lose weight?" My skinny jeans didn't make me look skinny anymore. My physician took a pause. "Maybe five pounds." I felt my face turn red, blushing. I was in between a time of squishing my now size 5 body into size 4 jeans. The doc blamed unwanted pounds on age-related slow-down of metabolism. I criticized the office scale. I vowed to do intermittent fasting (a diet cycle between a time of eating and fasting, which is healthy for some people).

The end result? I lost two pounds in one week. I agonized, "If I am going to cut back on calories, I'll do it with more flavor!" Enter herbs and spices to my gourmet rabbit food regimen of fresh fruits, vegetables, and whole grains. It worked. I dumped those five pesky pounds in one month.

DOCTOR'S ORDERS: SEASONINGS POUND PARING

Dr. Mehmet Oz, the well-known doctor on television, in one program discussed metabolism-boosting spices for weight loss. One of his picks included cayenne pepper. Dr. Ann Louise Gittleman, the popular health author of *Radical Metabolism*, also understands how herbs and spices help burning calories and weight loss. Take a look at some herbal weight loss wonders below. These seasonings are believed by nutritionists, doctors, and medical researchers to be a dieter's best friend.

8 FAT-BURNING HERBS AND SPICES

Cayenne: This hot spice can hike body temperature, which can spike metabolism. That means it is "thermogenic" meaning it ups body heat, which in turn can boost the metabolic rate. Some nutritionists believe it is calorie-burning. Read: After consuming it in food, you can burn dozens of calories at resting state.

Past research shows the ingredient capsaicin in cayenne is what gives the spice flavor and heat. If you're trying to burn calories, go ahead and savor a serving of salsa or put it in a soup or even on a southwestern omelet.

Often, if I want to drop a pound or two, I will use a cayenne salsa (homemade or store-bought) as a dressing for a kale salad mix. The heat of the spice satisfies my cravings for high fat food—and I feel satiated. But note, store-bought salsas do contain a lot of sodium so less is more—or make it yourself and 86 the salt.

Cardamom: Welcome to another thermogenic spice. Mix it up with other earthy flavored spices, including cloves and nutmeg. The autumn spice coffee I fell in love with contains the latter spices, and paired with a dash of cardamom it makes an aromatic and zesty brew. Plus, some studies believe the metabolism-boosting cardamom can give you energy to expend more calories. Caveat: It could also be the caffeine that provides that extra boost to get a move on.

Cloves: Diet guru Dr. Gittleman says, "Cloves are one of my unsung heroes for overall health and to rev up metabolism or calorie burning power." She points out, "As a parasite fighter, a pinch of cloves in your organic coffee or tea can help eliminate nutrient depleting hidden invaders." She recommends it's beneficial if you grind fresh cloves in a mortar pestle (the way you do cilantro for pesto) and brew, strain it for an herbal tea or coffee. Her words of wisdom made sense to me. Plus, after my five-pound weight gain wake-up call, I find it uncanny how before I knew the metabolism-boosting powers of cloves, I unwittingly purchased both specialty coffee and tea with cloves being one of the ingredients.

Cumin: One study has shown that cumin can help you burn up body fat. Nobody likes belly fat, whether you're a millennial, boomer, or in between. But cumin may come to the rescue. Here's proof: Iran researchers from the Shahid Sadoughi University of Medical Sciences conducted one study published in the *Complementary Therapies in Clinical Practice* journal. The study included eighty-eight obese and overweight women. One group consumed 1 teaspoon cumin added to yogurt twice a day for three months. The findings: There was improvement in weight, waist size, and a reduction in body fat percentage. A bonus: Cholesterol and triglycerides levels were improved, too.[1]

If adding cumin to foods can help you lose unwanted body fat, like it did in these women, it's worth trying 1 teaspoon each day to the dish of your choice.

Fennel: Dr. Gittleman also is a fan of fennel, the superhero herb used to help get rid of unwanted pounds. "Fennel is a wonderful herb to fight belly bloat and water retention that can pile on water weight," she explains. "Used as a tea from ready-made tea bags or in a shaved fennel bulb salad, this licorice tasting veggie is tops in my books on weight control." You can find fennel tea at grocery stores, health food stores, and online.

Fennel, A Medieval Appetite Suppressant

In researching fennel history, I discovered that British herbalist Nicholas Culpeper documented that parts of the fennel plant, including the seeds and leaves, are used in beverages. Drinks, like broth and tea, were slurped and sipped to help people slim down and healthy up. In medieval times, people believed fennel seeds helped suppress the appetite.

During past or present, the less you eat the more pounds you lose. In the film *The Devil Wears Prada*, one assistant at the magazine office admitted she ate nothing, only a cube of cheese if she felt faint. She did slim down to look model thin. However, drinking fennel tea, chewing fennel seeds, and adding fennel to a detox semi-fast could be more helpful in real life.

Parsley: This herb is a known diuretic, too. That means it can help you lose excess water weight. You may get that needed boost if starting a diet even if you gain the pounds back. Since it helps detox your body, it will provide that mental and temporary jump start needed to give you the incentive to lose unwanted weight.

Here is a detox savory and sweet parsley smoothie I whipped up that can be used year-round. In a blender, combine ½ cup fresh parsley (leaves and stems), 4 baby spinach leaves (pre-washed, packaged), ¾ cup fresh raspberries (fresh or frozen), 1 banana, sliced, 1 teaspoon cinnamon, ½ teaspoon cardamom, 1 teaspoon honey, and ¾ cup ice, crushed. Blend until smooth. Serves 2.

Saffron: A study published in the *Antioxidants* journal was conducted by researchers in Malaysia, who discovered saffron shows promise as an anti-obesity drug. The weight loss effect of saffron is unclear, but its ability to help lose weight includes providing satiety, the feeling of fullness due to the spike in brain chemicals or hormonal functions.[2]

Turmeric: Like cayenne, another fat-burning spice is this yellow colored one that has the ability to rev up your metabolism. Researchers give credit to curcumin, a primary compound in turmeric, that boosts heat, which like cayenne and cardamom may rev up a sluggish metabolism.

Skinny Herbal Popcorn for Chillaxing

Countless people, like me, and perhaps you, too, find themselves indulging in high-fat or sugary foods. Often stress is the enemy and eating a slice of cake or one too many cookies provides comfort. Well, popcorn comes to the rescue. This snack food is low-cal, low-fat, low-cholesterol, and it also contains calming vitamin B. Add herbs and spices and you've got a muncher's food that'll soothe frazzled nerves and fill you up not out.

Garlic and Parsley Popcorn

5 cups whole grain gourmet popped microwave popcorn
⅓ cup European-style butter (unsalted)
½ teaspoon garlic powder
½ teaspoon parsley, dried
½ teaspoon lemon pepper (Mountain Rose Herbs)
Pinch of sea salt
Parmesan cheese, shredded (for garnish)

In a large bowl, combine popcorn with a mixture of melted butter, garlic powder, parsley, lemon pepper, and salt. Sprinkle with cheese. Keep in sealed plastic container.

Serves 4.

This herb popcorn with a hint of butter, garlic, parsley, and pepper is satisfying and flavorful with its herbs and spices.

PEACE OUT, MINDLESS EATING

Ever notice when you gain extra unwanted pounds it's often due to emotions? Anxiety and stress can lead to mindless eating high-fat, high-calorie foods. So, I've put together a no-nonsense list of edibles, low-cal, low-fat stress busters—and paired them up with fat-burning herbs and spices. It's a win-win. Here, take a look and try a few on for size and watch your ideal size come back!

Apples: This crunchy, low-stress fruit fills you up and not out. It's rich in fiber, less than 100 calories, and sweet so it can satisfy unhealthy sugary cravings. Seasoning: Slice and sprinkle with allspice or cardamom or even calming nutmeg or cloves.

Baked Potato: Research has shown that eating complex carbs, like russet or sweet potatoes, can boost the brain chemical serotonin—it can calm frazzled nerves. Less than 150 calories, fiber-rich, and fat-free potatoes are a good weight loss food. Seasoning: Sprinkle with ground pepper, chives, and even a dash of cayenne.

Brown Rice: Another complex carb that is full of dietary fiber, and a half cup of brown rice is less than 100 calories and no fat. Seasoning: Mix in parsley and thyme. Or, get a big mix and add Mediterranean Blend.

Soup: A hot bowl of water-based soup with vegetables—not the creamy types—can calm you and fill you up, too. Seasoning: Mix in parsley, thyme, or herbs de Provence.

Water: Sipping H_2O often will keep you busy, hydrated, and fill you up replacing mindless eating. Add sprigs of parsley for flavor, color, and it is a diuretic to help you dump water weight giving you a jump start if you want to shed unwanted weight.

Pasta: Whole grain pasta provides a chill feel; it's rich in dietary fiber and not high in calories without a high-fat sauce. Seasoning: Add fennel or dill or try a spice blend like zaatar or Italian seasoning.

Popcorn: Seasoned popcorn without butter and salt can be diet-friendly. Instead of losing the low-cal, no-fat benefits, turn to herbs and spices to flavor up the crunch bites of goodness. Seasoning: Try sprinkling popcorn with allspice or pumpkin spice or a Mediterranean Blend for a savory flair.

No Diet Popcorn Recipes for Four Seasons

Popcorn is a good food for losing weight if you don't overdo butter. Less than more salt is preferred. It's adding seasonal herbs and spices that make it flavorful, crunchy, and a fun food to feed sugar, fat, and salt cravings. Here are four easy homemade recipes to get you started. You can easily mix and match combinations and enjoy each herby bite!

Autumn: Pumpkin Spice Nut Popcorn: 5 cups gourmet butter and sea salt popcorn, ¼ cup European-style butter (melted), ¼ cup honey, 1 teaspoon pumpkin spice, and ½ cup walnuts. Preheat the oven to 350 degrees F. In a large bowl, combine popped popcorn with a mixture of butter, honey, spice, and walnuts. Place on parchment-lined cookie sheet or pan. Bake for about 10 minutes. Turn a few times. When bubbly and toasted remove from oven. Cool. Keep in sealed container. The fridge is best.

Serves 4.

Winter: Herbes de Provence Popcorn: 5 cups whole grain popcorn, ¼ cup European-style butter (melted), ⅓ cup Parmesan cheese, shredded, 1 teaspoon herbes de Provence, 1 teaspoon thyme, and a dash of sea salt. In a large bowl, combine popped popcorn with mixture of butter, cheese, herbs, and salt. Turn a few times. Serve in a bowl.

Serves 4.

Spring: Lemon-Parsley Spicy Popcorn: 5 cups popcorn, ⅛ cup unsalted European-style butter (melted), 2 teaspoons parsley, dried, ½ teaspoon cayenne, ground, ½ teaspoon lemon pepper. In a large bowl, combine popped popcorn with mixture of butter, herbs, and spice. Serve in mini bowls.

Serves 4.

Summer: Caramel Cashew Lime Popcorn: 5 cups popcorn, ⅛ cup European-style butter (melted), ½ cup brown sugar, 2 teaspoons fresh lime juice, ½ cup cashews, ½ teaspoon sea salt. In a large bowl, combine butter and brown sugar, add juice. Mix in popcorn, nuts, and salt. Serve in bowl.

Serves 4.

TWO-DAY HERBAL INTERMITTENT FAST

Mini fasts (cutting calories but eating less as a jump-start diet) are nothing new. These days the two words "intermittent fasting" is a controversial trend. Medical doctors, like "Chasing Life" with Dr. Sanjay Gupta, CNN, said this type of diet can be healthful for some people. It may even boost longevity.

Before you start: Consult with your health practitioner. This plan isn't recommended for pregnant or nursing women, those with diabetes, high blood pressure, kidney problems, or anyone under age eighteen. Include fresh and dried herbs and spices that contrast with all the salty, fatty things you crave. Try allspice and nutmeg in soups, lemon and parsley in water, or dill in salads. Don't forget metabolism-boosting cayenne on vegetables and turmeric on rice. Take a multi-vitamin/mineral supplement daily. This two-day plan is only to be used for two days. You may repeat this two-day diet plan once a month. For this diet to work, do not consume more than 1200 calories per day.

Day 1

Water and lemon: Put fresh lemon juice in ice cube trays and freeze. Use two cubes in 12 ounces of water. Sprinkle with fresh parsley sprigs and a dash of cayenne.

Fruit juice: Blend your own juice using seasonal picks. Grapefruit is recommended.

Vegetable juice: Juice a ¼ cup each of kale, carrots, parsley, and cilantro.

Herbal tea: Try different varieties, including chamomile, cinnamon, dandelion, and thyme.

Vegetable broth: Use store-bought sodium type. Try a premium, organic brand.

1 cup water and lemon

Day 2

Breakfast: 1 cup fresh juice (grapefruit, preferred)

1 cup herbal tea

Lunch: 1 cup vegetable juice (store-bought or homemade)

1 cup brown rice, cooked

1 cup vegetables with herbs and spices

1 piece seasonal fruit

1 cup herbal tea

1 cup water, lemon and parsley sprigs

Dinner: 1 cup vegetable broth (low sodium) with 1 cup vegetables, herbs and spices

1 piece of fresh seasonal fruit

1 cup herbal tea

Slimming

Clove Stuffed Baked Apples

Back in the mid-twentieth century, we used whatever kind of apple we had on hand to bake apples. Baked apples were an autumn treat, often made during Halloween festivities. My mom served these apples to eat before trick-or-treating, so we'd be too full to eat all of the empty nutrition candy. Sweet and spicy apples can curb a sweet tooth. I changed it up a bit. I use Honeycrisp apples. Here's my European-style baked apples with a spicy twist.

2 Honeycrisp apples

DIVIDE FOR EACH APPLE:

2 tablespoons all-purpose flour
2 tablespoons brown sugar
    2 tablespoons European-style butter, melted
½ cup oats, uncooked
1 teaspoon cinnamon
¼ teaspoon cloves, ground
¼ teaspoon allspice
¼ teaspoon nutmeg
¼ cup pecans, chopped
¼ cup cranberries, dried
Cinnamon sticks and star anise for garnish (optional)

Preheat the oven to 350 degrees F. Rinse and cut apples in half. (Or you can slice tops off and bake them, too.) Scoop out seeds, making a hole. Set aside. In a bowl, combine flour, sugar, butter, oats, cinnamon, cloves, allspice, nutmeg, pecans, and cranberries. Stuff each apple crevice with the mixture. Place apples in a baking dish. Fill with 1 inch of water. Bake for 30 to 40 minutes or until tender. Serve right out of the oven. Top with a spoonful of vanilla ice cream. Drizzle with caramel sauce.

Serves 2.

So can herbs and spices help to stall Father Time? Yes! Anti-aging compounds in these timeless treasures can help add years to your life. Find out exactly how these gems are as good as gold and can be the secret of Super Agers.

HEALING HIGHLIGHTS FROM NATURE'S GARDEN-FEST

✓ Herbs and spices are epic wonders when you're dieting or want to maintain your weight. You won't miss fat, salt, and sugar—because seasonings give you satisfying flavor.

✓ Not only are herbs and spices low-calorie, low in fat and sodium, they're rich in antioxidants and nutrients . . . what you need when cutting calories and following portion control.

✓ Pairing low-fat fruits and vegetables flavored with fresh herbs and spices gives you extra nutritional benefits, too.

✓ More times than not, gourmet chefs use lots of fresh and dried herbs and spices. Why? Eating healthy is easier if you don't feel deprived of flavor.

✓ Indulge in a spicy, flavorful dish that beats a salty, fatty dish. (Think cold, fresh salsa seasoned with hot cayenne. Pair it with whole grain tortillas instead of processed potato chips.)

✓ Why not . . . sip water or herbal tea with fresh sprigs of parsley instead of a sugary soda or diet drink loaded with artificial sweeteners.

Longevity on the Rack

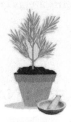

Thine eyes are sprigs in whose serene. And silent waters heaven is seen; Their lashes are the herbs that look On their young figures in the brook.
—WILLIAM C. BRYANT

I have memories of Saturdays with Molly, a centenarian. She was being cared for by my friend, the architect with a heart of gold who took me to the Indian restaurant. He kept his promise to take care of his mother if needed; he told me "till death do us part." One afternoon I said "yes" to staying with his bedridden mom and her senior Pomeranian. Her son cooked their favorite spicy dish from her recipe: Spicy Cioppino (without the shells and extra flavor). The gesture hit me (right) in the feels. The fish soup simmered on the stovetop. I could smell the garlic and thyme. I fed the woman the aromatic soup, spoonful by spoonful. She shared warmhearted stories of her son growing up on a small herb farm in Oregon. It was a day of herbal scents that fed her frail body and nourished my spirit—a tender memory.

ANTI-AGING HERBS AND SPICES

Today, age-defying baby boomers, like my neighbors next door, are often the caretakers of our parents who are living to be centenarians, like my architect friend's mom. And boomers, part of the graying of America, are adding years to their lives. We can give credit to good luck and good genes. And following a plant-centric clean foods diet is key to embracing the golden years.

Herbs and spices, fresh and dried, all varieties, can help turn back the clock and stall Father Time for a variety of reasons. Studies show seasonings contain antioxidants, which are anti-inflammatory, antiviral, and antibacterial—all qualities to keep health ailments and age-related diseases at bay. Because of the multiple specific isolated compounds, minerals, and vitamins in herbs and spices, they can help stall the aging process. Here, take a look at some age fighters that can help people to live a longer, healthier life.

FOREVER YOUNGER HERBS AND SPICES

Cardamom: It's believed adding a dash of cardamom to your diet can help regulate digestion and blood sugar levels. Some research shows this spice can enhance blood circulation. What's more, cardamom is touted for its stamina-providing benefits that keep us younger since we're more apt to keep moving.

Cilantro: The leaves and stems from the coriander plant can enhance a strong immune system. That in itself can keep colds and flu at bay. Also, bolstering your immunity with cilantro can also keep you well so you lower the risk of viral infections. If you don't fall victim to pneumonia or a super bug, your life span is going to be extended.

Cardamom: This spice can keep your blood sugar levels steady, which can keep diabetes away. Cardamom also boosts living a longer life by its ability to keep your blood circulation healthy and enhance physical energy.

Cayenne: The compound capsaicin, an inflammatory used to lessen joint pain, can help you stay physically active. We know regular exercise can aid in keeping our heart healthier, and even stave off chronic ailments, such as depression to even cancer.

Cloves: Rich in antioxidants, like eugenol, this spice can help stall Father Time by keeping the body's cells healthy. Also, it is helps to block blood platelets, and keep our arteries unclogged, lessening the odds of heart attack or stroke.

Garlic: This popular heart-healthy herb is known by medical researchers to help lower bad cholesterol and blood pressure. Heart disease is still the number one killer in America, and adding garlic to your diet may lower the risk of developing cardiovascular problems. Studies also show garlic can help keep blood sugar levels on an even keel and stave off diabetes.

A friend of mine, a retired physical therapist in her seventies, was married to a busy attorney. We used to swim together, talk about food, and her hardheaded husband. One night the health-oriented woman served spaghetti. Instead of hamburger she substituted the meat with turkey. Her mate of fifty years asked, "What did you do to this dish?" She told him the truth as he refused to eat the repurposed recipe. A few weeks later, she used half beef and half turkey. This time she added garlic and herbes de Provence in the marinara sauce. He raved about the herbal spaghetti that was the best EVER. She outsmarted her mate and the couple lived full, energetic lives throughout their eighties.

Oregano: Another Mediterranean herb, oregano contains immune-boosting compounds to fight germs and inflammation.

Turmeric: An Indian favorite in cuisine, turmeric also is an age-fighting antioxidant, anti-inflammatory spice. Not only does it contain anti-cancer compounds, but it's a heart-healthy spice, too, thanks to curcumin, which unclogs your arteries. That means less odds of developing heart attacks and strokes. Also, as we are an aging society because people are living longer, turmeric helps guard the brain; it can help keep memory to dementia at bay.

Anti-Arthritis and the Garlic Helper

One Thanksgiving dinner, I recall my ex-mate's older sister who didn't like me asking a sobering question while I munched on the turkey stuffing with bits of garlic: "How will you survive if you get arthritis? How will you write?" I didn't answer the question but got flashes of reading about Henry James. Once stricken by pain, stiffness, swelling in his hands, he hired a transcriptionist and wrote verbally. That scenario spooked me as did her snipes about me being too thin as I ate a second helping of garlicky stuffing.

Years later, an author comrade stopped writing because of rheumatoid arthritis, which did affect his hands. Also, at the same time, I witnessed a sixty-something neighbor slow down due to osteoarthritis. As time passed, I never was stricken by arthritis in my hands or body, but I did fear losing my writer hands (or my brain) like a character in a doctor show where they are stricken by a disease that affects their lifestyle.

In real life, 50 million American adults are affected by arthritis. It is more common in women than men. Also, genes, previous joint injury, and old age play a role. The important thing is to lessen pain and guard your joints. Herbalists believe some herbs and spice can help control arthritis, too.

Enter garlic. As noted, it is a popular herb for health and it can help fight arthritis pain and swelling. Past research, in the lab and with humans, shows fresh garlic can stall pro-inflammatory substances called cytokines. Researchers at King's College London and the University of East Anglia conducted a study on how garlic may protect against hip osteoarthritis. Their findings, published in the *BMC Musculo-skeletal Disorders* journal, show the compounds found in garlic are key. The UK scientists discovered that women who eat a diet rich in fruit and vegetables, especially alliums like garlic, were less likely to develop arthritis in the hip joint. Credit is given to a compound called diallyl disulfide, which inhibits cartilage-damaging enzymes when introduced to a human cartilage cell-line in the lab. More research is needed but the research shows promise.[1]

Try eating 1 garlic clove per day. Do consult with your health practitioner before you start.

THINK YOUNG ABOUT HERBS AND SPICES

Adopt New Seasonings: Ever notice how some people seem to have tunnel vision when it comes to using herbs and spices? In other words, they refuse to see other seasonings. This, in turn, can result in boredom.

Adding new herbs and spices to your daily regimen can refresh your recipes—food, home cures, and beauty. Try something new and grow your garden of seasonings for the thrill of it. You may be pleasantly surprised.

Use Happy Herbs and Spices: Turn to the seasonings that contain compounds that can up those feel-good hormones, like serotonin and dopamine. These happy seasonings are essential during wintertime when there is a lack of sunshine. Also, happy herbs and spices can boost your mood if you're feeling a bit under the weather.

Seek Help: Let's face it, nobody is a know-all seasonings guru. Things change. If you try a new herb or spice and it doesn't seem to pan out—patience! Seek an herbalist, health food store worker, or pharmacist.

You may not be using the herb or spice the right way for you. Or perhaps you're using too little, too late or maybe the wrong form.

Find a Healing Herb and Spice Goal: So, what is your purpose? Are you using herbs and spices to spice up your meals? Or is it your goal to supplement your diet with an herb or spice or a mix to beat an ailment. Find out what your intentions are, then follow your instincts for best results. Remember: No one herb or spice fits all.

HERBS AND SPICES KEEP YOU AFLOAT (AT ANY AGE)

I've shared with you Dr. Will Clower, the modern-day seafarer who fearlessly sails with wife Dottie—and herbs and spices are part of the adventures. As I entered my expedition into the land of plant therapy, he simultaneously was riding the swells and squalls from sea to sea. Here, take a look below at his candid journal entry. He wrote his words in present tense (like you do writing in a diary). This entry was created before he landed ashore in the America on the East Coast, after his first trip around the world . . .

TRANSATLANTIC DAY 14: HE ATE MY PLANT!

We'll be back on land in two days, with cars and malls and all the normal stuff that normal people have and do every day. We were normal once. Had the house, the car, and the garden in a few different cities like Atlanta, Pittsburgh, Syracuse, and Raleigh. Of all the things about "normal," I miss the plants and herbs the most. We had the most amazing sage plant, woody and robust with leaves just begging to go into your baked chicken. At the risk of sounding like a Paul Simon song, yes, we had "parsley sage rosemary and thyme" to go with our tomatoes and basil that grew so huge in the summer we swore it was some kind of mutant plant from *Little Shop of Horrors*.

HOW *AMARI* GOT PLANTS

So, when we strolled through the Carrefour in Cartagena, Spain, and Dottie saw potting soil, it was like someone had cast a spell over my wife, with an almost trancelike voice and that far away stare. Remember dirt? Mmmm, I want to put my fingers in it . . . we have to get some! Her mind, now feverish with uncontrolled gardenlust, started scanning the shelves like a junkie in need of a hit.

"We need pots," she intoned. To which I replied, "You do know we live on a B. O. A. T., right? On the water?" She didn't respond to my question, confirming both its irrelevance and her need to find a plant pusher. "Just a couple," she said.

Then it happened. She eyed the plant section. Her movement slowed somewhat as she edged forward, like she didn't want to startle them on approach.

"Hey, look at this one," she said pointing to a nice healthy basil plant. I held that basil and it looked right back at me with those beautiful green leaves. And like kittens, once you pick them up, they are yours. Unlike kittens I suppose, I'm thinking about chopping these up and throwing them into my food: Caprese salad and pasta sauces . . .

Next was the mint plant, which instantly gave me religious visions of mojitos accompanied by choirs of angels singing the Hallelujah Chorus! And aww, look at the cute little woody rosemary plant that we could take home, chop up and put into white bean dip.

Is it a garden? No, not so much. Have I gotten mojito 1 out of little mister mint? Nope and likely will never. But adding these plants to *Amari*'s cockpit does two important things. It gives a little green splash of color that reminds us both of growing things. But also, it's like aroma therapy—whenever you pass your hand over them you get that fresh mint, almost anise-like fragrance from the basil, and that earthy rosemary.

THE NEAR-DEATH EXPERIENCE

So typically, on the SV *Amari* when morning happens, coffee quickly follows, then we go up into the cockpit to welcome the day and to slowly ease our brains back on line. Job one is to give our babies just a little water, to get them through the warm and sunny day in the cockpit. That's when Dottie saw it. The mint plant was demolished! Practically denuded! Something had chewed up most of the leaves. How could this happen? Then we saw him. An inch worm, right there brazenly lingering on one of the few remaining twigs of my mint plant! There he was all plump after his gorge fest all-nighter, still morning-drunk on my mint no doubt.

Little worm ate my plant. I'm not sure how he thought his day was going to go, but he suddenly found himself in the ocean. No doubt some fish gobbled him up and thought, mmm minty fresh! Anyway, no need to send cards, flowers, and get-well balloons, the mint plant has made a full recovery and is doing well. The inch worm, not so much.

TALES OF A GALLEY SLAVE

Two dinners left to make on this passage. We have a ton of meat in the freezer, but just enough fresh stuff to eek out one last Greek salad with tomatoes, cucumber, onion, feta and black olives. The baby red potatoes were also a big hit last time and there were a couple of those rolling around in the cabinet. And we figured that the chicken will need to be eaten before the pork, so thighs it is. Great, so. Thighs. With what? That's the issue. I can put them in the oven on their own to dry out into shoe leather, but they're telling me that they really want a sauce or something.

So, while pondering these mysteries, I bought myself some time by tossing oil in a pan. "That pan looks like it wants some garlic." And later it added that it wanted some chili flakes for heat, and oregano because it just feels like it's turning into a Mediterranean kind of thing tonight. Glancing in the cupboard, oh look, sun-dried tomatoes. That'll work with my new theme!! And for the liquid needed in the pan to keep them moist, I poured in the remaining red wine from my glass and mixed it through. I kept the lid on to keep the fluids brewing until the very end. It turned out to be quite delicious, and the crew was well satisfied.

Tomorrow is our last meal on the transatlantic passage, and I'm not sure what's on that menu just yet. But who knows, maybe I'll graze past the herbs and get a whiff of inspiration that may land us in Asia, Thailand, or France. World travel, *Amari* style.

So, plants—herbs and spices—have a place on land or sea—and in your life wherever you are. Also, eating the Mediterranean diet (remember herbs and spices included in the pyramid) and abiding by the lax Mediterranean lifestyle, the way Europeans do—can keep you younger in mind and body. Research shows Europeans live longer lives, have less heart disease than Americans, and often are leaner. They eat good colorful food enhanced with a garden-variety of herbs and spices.

Age-Defying

No Shells Garlic Cioppino

This West Coast fish dish is a favorite of mine since my mom first served it to me. I've enjoyed it with folks in their 70s, 80s, 90s, and beyond—like the architect's mom. It is a soup with anti-aging garlic, fennel, bay leaf, fish, tomatoes, and wine. This recipe is my creation, inspired by the people in my life who have aged gracefully, and have forever left an imprint on my mind and soul.

¼ cup olive oil
1 onion
1 large fennel bulb, sliced
4 garlic cloves, chopped
4 cups fresh tomatoes
1 cup white wine
4 tablespoons tomato paste
Sea salt and ground pepper to taste
1 teaspoon herbes de Provence
1 bay leaf
1 cup fresh parsley, chopped
½ pound halibut, cut in 1 inch cubes
1 pound crab
1 pound shrimp
½ pound scallops

In a large pot add oil, onions, fennel, and garlic. Cook over medium heat until soft. Add tomatoes, wine, tomato paste, salt, pepper, herbes de Provence, and bay leaf. Simmer for 15 minutes covered, add parsley. Add halibut and cook about 5 minutes. Add remaining seafood, cook covered 5 minutes. Remove bay leaf.

Serves 12.

Pair with fresh, soft baguette and European-style butter.

It's time. It's time to share the savvy and special ways—some to be used internally and others topically—you can put herbs and spices to work for home cures. That's right, DIY home folk remedies.

HEALING HIGHLIGHTS FROM NATURE'S GARDEN-FEST

✓ Herbs and spices are twenty-first century because of their components that help stall aging and infuse food with nature's goodness.

✓ Plant-based diets teamed with herbs and spices are key to longevity.

✓ By using herbs and spices with fruits and vegetables, and whole grains, it adds aroma, flavor, and disease-fighting antioxidants to guard against age-related diseases.

✓ One herb or one spice is not a magic cure-all to age-related diseases. Mix it up to get more anti-aging nutrients.

✓ But, adding a specific herb like garlic or spice like turmeric with a healthy diet and lifestyle may be just what the doctor ordered—or one day in the future will do just that!

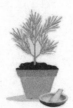

PART 4

FOLK REMEDIES

Herbal Healings from the Garden

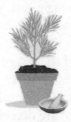

Time is an herb that cures all Diseases.
—BENJAMIN FRANKLIN

On a mid-autumn day I turned to spice to get me through the noise challenge of getting a new roof. I sipped chamomile tea spiked with allspice. It calmed my nerves. The store-bought anise cookies helped boost my mood and repeat like my gran taught me to say, "This too shall pass."

In the late afternoon, I believe the herb-infused hot chocolate I sipped was a gift of feeling chill. The new roof was completed in one day, the dog rescued from the kennel before 6:00 P.M. It was done. We survived the event. To this day I give credit to the wonder of calming herbs and spices.

I'm sharing dozens of tried-and-true home cures using herbs and spices to help deal with common health ailments. I'll discuss the ailment, remedy prescription, and why it works. Nutmeg for acne? Black pepper for a cough? Parsley for bloat? Yes! You'll be amazed to discover how each of these herbs and spices can be used topically or consumed and put to work in many ways. Sometimes, Mother Nature knows best. Read on.

DIY CURE #1: GOT ANXIETY? CHILL WITH ALLSPICE

Stress overload is often a trigger for high anxiety, slamming the nervous system on overdrive. Most people will feel anxious, sooner or later. Going to the dentist, taking a test, waiting for an important letter or check to arrive can wreak havoc on your brain and body. That means worrying to falling into the "what if?" trap, feeling edgy, irritable, and distracted are some of the symptoms that'll pay you a visit.

General anxiety disorder (GAD) hangs around like a friend that overstays their welcome. (Note: That is three days, according to Benjamin Franklin.) Folks who are diagnosed with GAD, like me, instead of staying in the moment, fast-forward to the future. I use the "what if?" catastrophic thinking chip in my brain. Worrying about things you cannot control can cause a racing heart, feeling on edge, and simply feeling out of sync with reality. But allspice can come to your rescue!

What Herbal Rx to Use: Put a dash of allspice in a 12-ounce cup of chamomile tea. Savor the moment. Sip a cuppa of the spicy brew. Repeat as needed.

Why Spicing It Up Works: Allspice is a mixture of calming compounds. It contains anti-inflammatory ingredients that can quell pain. If you have a headache or backache, for instance, it can trigger stress, and anxiety may follow. Once the inflammation is lessened, however, a sense of centeredness may be the end result. It is comforting in a cup of milk or coffee and/or if infused in a warm cinnamon roll or creamy rice pudding.

DIY CURE #2: BAD BREATH? PARSLEY PLEASE

Halitosis is not a sweet thing. The good news is, there is a home remedy for it. Often, an odor in the mouth can be due to a sinus problem, not drinking enough water, or eating a pungent-smelling food. Parsley can come to the rescue.

What Herbal Rx to Use: Ready-to-drink green juices including the herb parsley are convenient? These beverages in a bottle are available at grocery stores and Whole Foods Market. But you can whip up a DIY drink, too. Parsley Beverage: 1 apple, 1/2 cup parsley, fresh (all of the herb), 2 tablespoons raw honey. Combine in a blender and juice it. Serves 1.

Why Spicing It Up Works: Drinking parsley juice, much like munching on a sprig of parsley, works to freshen breath. How? The chlorophyll (absorbent green pigments in green plants) in the green, leafy herb soaks up the bad odor in your mouth. If the cause is acute from a garlic dish or seasonal allergies on a day when the pollen or ragweed is high, it's your remedy. But note, if you have a dental problem, such as a cavity, leaky filling, or gingivitis, make a dental appointment.

DIY CURE #3: FEELING BLOATED? DEFLATE WITH DILL

Bloating is when your tummy is full of liquid or gas. It can feel puffy and make you feel uncomfortable. It's a problem that can blindside you and make not zippering your jeans seem minor in contrast to the discomfort. Causes include hormones (during PMS to menopause), eating too much fiber (35 to 50 grams per day is normal), drinking carbonated beverages, chewing gum, and even swallowing air due to stress and anxiety. Try a folk remedy to help you get that flatter stomach and feel normal.

What Herbal Rx to Use: Enter dill. Dill tastes like "parsley with personality" and it "acts like a natural diuretic and relieves intestinal bloating," explains popular nutritionist and author Dr. Ann Louise Gittleman. She uses it on plain yogurt to salads. "It's tangy and cooling." Adds Gittleman: "I use it on lamb chops." Before serving the dish, she will sprinkle fresh chopped dill on top of the lean protein.

Why Spicing It Up Works: Natural diuretics get rid of water weight that can give you a bloat. It helps to balance sodium and potassium. One trip to Southern California in a huge RV is a vacation I'd like to forget. I left with an over-the-counter bloat medicine. It didn't help. When coming back home on a Friday evening on the busy freeway it caused bloat with a capital B. I ended up finally getting off the interstate and took a break at a restaurant. A waitress suggested putting strained dill seeds in a cup of hot tea. I did it later on the journey and give credit to her dill Rx.

DIY CURE #4: BLOOD CLOTS? GARLIC TO UNCLOG ARTERIES

A stroke happens when a blood vessel in your brain ruptures. It is not an epic event you ever want to experience. When I was a working grad student, one morning I arrived at a house-cleaning job. The homeowner's elderly mother was pet sitting. I sensed she was a bit off. "My head hurts," she repeated. On the stairs my eyes saw shattered glass-framed photos. I assumed she had fallen down the steps and I told my boss. One week later: A major stroke followed.

You are more at risk of blood clots if your blood is sticky and blocks your arteries from good circulation. It is no secret that if you have high blood pressure, you may be more at risk of a hemorrhagic stroke because the walls of your blood vessels may be prone to a clot or blockage. A clove of garlic (or a bit from one), according to herbal folklore, helps your blood from becoming sticky and can help unclog arteries, lessening the odds of blood clots. Yes, consumed regularly it can help thin your blood paired with nature's foods, including fish also part of the Mediterranean diet.

What Herbal Rx to Use: Take one clove of a garlic a day. You can consume it raw or add it to food, such as pizza, stew, soup, or even eat it raw. Or try taking a garlic capsule. Follow directions on the right amount for you.

Why Spicing It Up Works: Garlic is a natural blood thinner and may keep your blood running smoothly like water from the tap without any clogs. I recall an octogenarian friend who told me after he had a mini stroke, the doctors put him on warfarin. Not knowing what it was I soon discovered it was a blood thinner. Scientific studies show adding garlic to your diet can help thin the blood and perhaps lower the risk of blood clots.

Safety Sound Bite: If you are taking a prescription blood thinner, however, it is strongly advised not to take garlic. Why? Blood thinning medications or aspirin and garlic can have an adverse reaction because it could result in unmanageable bleeding.

DIY CURE #5: HIT WITH A BRUISE?
LOSE IT WITH PARSLEY

A bruise is an injury showing in a region of discolored skin on the body. It can happen by an accidental impact rupturing blood vessels. We've all experienced a bruise or two in life. The last bruise I endured was when my former Brittany spaniel–excited puppy lunged at my face. Blindsided by his paws and nails, I ended up going to the E.R. for stitches. I asked the nurse, "Will it scar?" No answer. Hours later, the red and swollen skin above my upper lip began to discolor and turn black and blue. Ice was my home remedy. But there was another home cure for bruising I learned about later.

What Herbal Rx to Use: Use fresh or dried parsley mixed in a half-and-half ratio with olive oil. Make a smooth paste. Apply the parsley goop to the bruise. Repeat 2 to 3 times per day.

Why Spicing It Up Works: A versatile herb like parsley contains anti-inflammatory compounds as does antioxidant-rich olive oil. Also, parsley boasts vitamin K, which can lessen a sore and swollen bruise. If you have a deficiency of this blood-clotting vitamin you may be more prone to bruising. So not only use it topically when a bruise happens but as a preventive herb by tossing it into your diet regime. (Unfortunately, I do have a small scar and parsley isn't a miracle cure.)

DIY CURE #6: DOWN WITH A COLD? GARLIC HAS GOT THIS

A common cold is a nuisance. It's like an unwanted visitor that intrudes in your life, especially during the wintertime. Also, when traveling via plane, train, or even a car with people a cold is contagious. The telltale sore throat, sneezing, and sniffles signify the cold virus. The upside: You can bolster your immune system to guard against catching the bug and to keep you well.

What Herbal Rx to Use: Mix 1 tablespoon fresh garlic, minced with ½ cup vegetables. Stir-fry. Repeat twice a day during a cold outbreak and before traveling.

Why Spicing It Up Works: Garlic is packed with antiviral properties that enhance the immune system, and that may keep you cold-free. What's more, including garlic in your daily diet, whether it's sipping an herbal soup, tea, or even taking a supplement, can prevent you from catching future colds no matter where you go or what season it is.

DIY CURE #7: FEELING CONGESTED? DRY OUT WITH CAYENNE

Seasonal allergies can be miserable for countless people. Certain allergens, including pollen and ragweed, can affect your nose and throat. Sneezing? Sniffling? Scratchy throat? You've entered the land of culprits that can cause nasal congestion. During the summer, fall, and spring I go online and track the allergy chart; it's sort of like a weather forecast. You type in your city and state, and it will rank the level of allergens! Achoo! Seriously, if ragweed ranks high, I bring out my arsenal of nature's cures.

What Herbal Rx to Use: Include cayenne, dried and ground or fresh and chopped in food, such as salsa or in a salad. Use once or twice per day. Or take cayenne pepper in capsule form once a day as needed. Also, try ¼ teaspoon of cayenne pepper powder mixed in 1 cup of black tea.

Why Spicing It Up Works: Research studies have shown hot and spicy foods can rev up blood circulation. This, in result, is like a humidifier; it can help open clogged and inflamed nasal passages and you may breathe easier. The heat of the herbal remedy may help sinus infections, too.

A study published in the journal *Annals of Allergy, Asthma & Immunology* gives credit to a nasal spray containing the capsaicin compound. Researchers at the University of Cincinnati Academic Health Center discovered heat in chili peppers fight inflammation and can ease sinus congestion, sniffles, and postnasal drip.[1]

I can personally attest whipping up a spicy and hot homemade salsa or using a fresh store-bought variety—including cayenne—does its job. Instantly, I feel like my nose isn't as stuffy. It clears the sinuses so a headache between the eyes often goes away. Paired with drinking plenty of water this trick from nature works wonders.

Kick a Virus with Herbes de Provence

Remember in your childhood when you weathered a bout of a cold or flu? It's likely your mama helped you to feel better by serving up a dish of hot soup with a mix of herbs. It could have been canned or homemade. As long as there was a combination of herbs in the broth it helped the symptoms of congestion.

Try eating an 8-ounce cup or bowl of hot herbal chicken soup with 1 teaspoon herbes de Provence. It can be homemade or canned. Repeat 2 times daily. Doctors know chicken soup can lessen mucus and reduce congestion, which often comes with seasonal allergies, cold, and flu. Spices, including cayenne and garlic, contain anti-inflammatory and antibacterial compounds that work to break down the goo in your throat. Herbes de Provence is a mix of dried herbs from France. It can contain thyme, which is known to help aid mucus in the throat.

Provencal Chicken Soup

❖ ❖ ❖

1 cup onion, diced
1 cup celery, sliced
1 cup carrots, sliced
3 tablespoons Pasolivo Lemon Olive Oil
1 tablespoon Pasolivo Pacific Blue Kosher Sea Salt
Pasolivo Lavender Spice Blend
1 tablespoon Pasolivo herbes de Provence
32 ounces chicken broth
1 cup zucchini, sliced
1 (15-ounce) can diced or sliced tomatoes
2 to 4 chicken thighs, boneless skinless, diced bite-size
½ cup barley or brown rice (optional)
3 tablespoons Pasolivo Lemon Olive Oil, to finish
2 tablespoons chopped parsley to finish (optional)

In a large Dutch oven or stock pot (minimum 4 quart), on medium-high heat, sauté onion, celery, and carrots in Pasolivo Lemon Olive Oil with Pasolivo Pacific Blue Kosher Sea Salt and Pasolivo Lavender Spice Blend until tender, about 4–7 minutes. Stirring to avoid burning, but not too often so the vegetables will start to caramelize. Lower heat to medium-low and add remaining ingredients, except 3 tablespoons Pasolivo Lemon Olive Oil and chopped parsley (optional) for finishing. Stir to combine and bring to a simmer. Once simmering, reduce heat and simmer until barley or brown rice are tender (about 40 minutes). If serving right away, drizzle with remaining 3 tablespoons Lemon Olive Oil and sprinkle chopped parsley (optional). Taste for seasoning and serve. Otherwise, let sit until cool and refrigerate or freeze. Reheat when ready to serve.

Yield: 8 cups.

(Courtesy: Pasolivo)

DIY CURE #8: EEW! CONJUNCTIVITIS?
DUMP IT WITH CILANTRO

Eye doctors will tell you that infections that can be caused by viruses or bacteria can end up as pink eye aka "conjunctivitis." Simply put, it is an inflammation of the conjunctivas of the eyes and makes the eyes red. There can be discharge and it can also burn. Rubbing your eyes will worsen the ailment. You can try a home remedy to heal a mild case or until you see a health practitioner or eye doctor.

What Herbal Rx to Use: Combine ¼ cup cilantro leaves with ¼ cup water. Strain the liquid. Apply the wet pulp of cilantro leaves on your closed eyelids. Leave on for about 5 or 10 minutes 2 times per day.

Why Spicing It Up Works: Medical studies have shown it is the essential oils in cilantro that have antibacterial action. Plus, anti-inflammatory compounds in cilantro offer a soothing effect to skin irritations. When I was a teenager, one of the toddlers I babysat had the contagious pink eye. I used the cilantro home remedy on my eyelids as a preventive treatment. I thought it was odd putting green goop on my eyelids, but as a self-professed hypochondriac I didn't want to contract the eye problem. And I didn't.

DIY CURE #9: UGH! CONSTIPATED?
GET GOING WITH FENNEL

Welcome to irregularity: The consensus of medical doctors is, if you are having less than three bowel movements a week, constipation is part of your life. Nobody is immune to the constipation blues. It can be triggered by many things, including not drinking enough water, not eating enough dietary fiber, being too sedentary, and traveling, which comes with change in routine. Getting back on track isn't rocket science. Enter the right herb to help get your bathroom groove back.

What Herbal Rx to Use: Put 1 teaspoon roasted fennel seeds in an 8-ounce cup of hot water. Steep and strain. Add lemon juice to taste. Drink the fennel-lemon tea before bedtime.

Why Spicing It Up Works: Fennel can get the digestion process back in running order, so to speak. How? How does it do it? It can unclog your plumbing by making gastric enzymes to help get rid of waste. Also, water and lemon are known to be natural aids for getting and staying regular.

DIY Cure #10: Got a Cough?
Halt It with Cardamom

Ever notice after a bad cold an annoying cough follows? Or if you have seasonal allergies, thanks to pollen or ragweed, a cough can be a bother. Want to stop the annoying tickle? Instead of trying a yucky-tasting over-the-counter cough syrup or sugary lozenge (I chipped a lower molar on one of those hard-medicinal candies, much like the dried fig incident), why not try sipping tea? Turn to your spice rack and grab tea leaves or a bag to help halt that coughing faster than you can say "cough."

What Herbal Rx to Use: Add a dash of cardamom powder in an 8-ounce cup of tea. Black or green tea is best because of the double dose of antioxidants. Chamomile brew is good, too. Add a bit of honey if you prefer a sweeter flavor. When I endured a cough from seasonal allergies, I substituted cardamom with 1 teaspoon of dried thyme in a cup of hot water. I steeped the herb, drained it, and added honey to the brew.

Why Spicing It Up Works: Cardamom boasts anti-inflammatory compounds. When you consume the ground spice it can help quell the tickle in your throat. Well, that is the theory. Due to allergens from my double-dense-coat Australian shepherd and sinusitis, I gave the cardamom and tea remedy a go. After sipping a cup of the anti-cough cure, I was cough-free. A bonus: After the tooth chip and a one-thousand-dollar crown, my cough cure is cardamom and tea.

DIY CURE #11: CUTS AND PUNCTURES? GARLIC IS ON IT

Ouch! Imagine you get a superficial cut or wound on your skin. After the initial shock of the accident, reality sets in. It hurts. First and foremost, you want to stop the bleeding. Then, you begin to think about guarding the wound against infection. After washing the cut, disinfecting it with an antibacterial remedy, like soap and peroxide, you'll want to keep your skin clean. Then, nature's antibiotic comes to the rescue.

What Herbal Rx to Use: Combine 3 garlic cloves, crushed with 1 cup apple cider vinegar. Apply to the cut 3 times per day.

Why Spicing It Up Works: Garlic contains the compound allicin, which has both antibacterial and anti-fungal properties. The combination of garlic and vinegar, another natural antibacterial superfood, can fight germs and guard against infection. As a dog person, I admit at least twice when my canines were in their first year, they were full of energy. The latest incident, my Australian shepherd's nail swiped my face. I dodged an infection by using vinegar, but next time I will combine it with garlic for an extra ounce of protection.

DIY CURE #12: EARACHE PAIN? BABY 'EM WITH TURMERIC

If you do not have too much wax, an ear infection, or perforated eardrum, you are lucky. Also, during or after a flight your ears may ache due to the changes in cabin pressure and altitude—made worse if you're congested. If it is a minor earache and/or you are waiting to see a doctor, an herbal treatment may be helpful.

What Herbal Rx to Use: Combine ¼ teaspoon turmeric powder with ¼ teaspoon echinacea. Add the antibiotic herbs into 8 ounces of hot water. Steep for 3 minutes. Add ½ teaspoon of honey. Repeat a few times per day, preferably as a preventive measure before an upcoming event that could trigger an earache.

Why Spicing It Up Works: Both herbs have antibiotic and antiseptic compounds. Not only can a super herbal duo fight a potential ear infection, but it may prevent it. Also, while you are waiting for the herbs to do their job, applying a warm heating pad on your ear(s) can help lessen any inflammation and diminish the pain. On a flight from Honolulu to San Francisco I recall during the landing that it affected both my ears. Not only did I hear babies on the aircraft crying, but I complained to my traveling companion. "My ears hurt!" He said, "You should have taken turmeric and echinacea. I told you." He was not in pain. And it was an "aha" moment that maybe his herbal remedy could be helpful for a future flight.

DIY CURE #13: GOT A FEVER?
COOL DOWN WITH CILANTRO

A fever can pay you a visit before coming down with the flu or even pneumonia. A fever is a part of the body's disease-fighting power. When the body temperature rises it is killing off disease-producing organisms. Symptoms of a fever may include muscle aches, feeling warmish, a headache, chills, and weakness. A normal temperature is 98.6 degrees F. If you feel like you have a fever, take your temperature and if it is 100 degrees F you may be able to take control and bring it down with an herbal remedy.

What Herbal Rx to Use: In a blender, combine ⅛ cup of fresh cilantro leaves with ½ cup of water. Blend until smooth. Strain the pulp. Take 2 teaspoons of the cilantro juice a few times per day.

Why Spicing It Up Works: Cilantro juice is a popular folk remedy. It is chock-full of antioxidants and flavonoids that are immune-boosting. Also, cilantro contains chlorophyll, which helps detoxify the body of toxins; this can enhance your immune system and help you fight an onset of a fever. One trip returning from Canada and laid over in Seattle, a fever haunted me in my hotel room. I felt like the *Contagion* character calling up her boss to tell him of her illness. Instead, I called the airline and rebooked my flight so I could get a few extra hours of sleep and stay hydrated. If I knew about the cilantro juice remedy, I would have called room service. Instead, I made green tea.

DIY CURE #14: FIBROMYALGIA STIFFNESS?
LOOSEN UP WITH CAYENNE

Aches and pains in the body could be a sign of fibromyalgia. Decades ago, doctors didn't believe it was a real disorder. As time passed, fibromyalgia has been defined as a health condition. There is even a prescription medication to help symptoms. However, if you have flare-ups or are uncertain if you even have it, you can turn to herbalism for relief.

What Herbal Rx to Use: Try using a topical cream with cayenne's compound capsaicin. Apply the cream as needed.

Why Spicing It Up Works: Cayenne contains capsaicin, which is an ingredient in topical pain-relieving capsaicin cream available over the counter at pharmacies. It works to lessen muscle aches and pains. My personal remedy during the colder months in autumn and winter, which can trigger a flare-up, is as follows: I swim in an indoor swimming pool, and then soak in a hot tub. Once home if I am bothered by aching arms or legs from walking the dog in the snow or bringing in firewood, I will use the capsaicin cream on my achy-breaky upper back or lower back.

DIY CURE #15: BEARING FLATULENCE?
GET YOUR FENNEL FIX

Not only is gas in the stomach and bowels disturbing, it can be uncomfortable. One time at a theater, I bought a coffee. Within twenty minutes after drinking the beverage, distention of my belly and discomfort along with gas occurred. I spent the entire time in the bathroom. Perhaps I couldn't have stopped this unfortunate happening, but if flatulence pays you an untimely visit there is a home remedy to consider.

What Herbal Rx to Use: After a meal, chew ½ teaspoon of fennel seeds. Use a chaser of about ½ cup of water.

Why Spicing It Up Works: Fennel is touted for its compounds that act as a digestive aid and for good reason. Fennel seeds contain antibacterial and anti-inflammatory properties that help to eliminate the bacteria that causes gassiness or an upset stomach. The seeds can relieve inflammation and irritation in the intestines by soothing muscles to relieve gas. After the movie mishap of stomach distress, I discovered by talking with the coffee vendor that the coffee carafe wasn't washed properly, and the residue may have been the culprit.

DIY CURE #16: FLU BUG? SCRATCH IT WITH CAYENNE

Influenza is a bug that nobody wants to catch. During the fall and winter months is the time when the flu bug seems to be more prevalent. Perhaps it is due to being indoors more and closer to people who may be infected. If your immune system is compromised you may be prone to contracting the virus.

What Herbal Rx to Use: Try the Anti-Flu Cocktail, created by Bill Gottlieb, Certified Health Coach. Put together a pinch of cayenne, 1 or 2 cloves of garlic, 3 droppers of echinacea tincture, 3 droppers of goldenseal tincture, 3 droppers of cat's claw tincture, the juice of half a lemon, and 6 to 8 ounces of vegetable juice. Drink twice a day whenever you feel like you may be coming down with the flu.

Why Spicing It Up Works: *Alternative Cures* author Gottlieb of Trinidad, California, gives kudos to his favorite wintertime Anti-Flu Cocktail. He touts cayenne pepper with its active ingredient, capsaicin. "Studies show capsaicin provides lots of other benefits aside from beefing up my immune system," he points out.

Free Falling! Cabin Fever Herbs

Cabin fever? It is real. Feeling irritable? Restless? Isolation or confined indoors for too long can cause you to be as nervous as a cat. Turn to tarragon and thyme. Tarragon contains eugenol, known to help relieve anxiety. Sprinkle the herb on a bowl of soup or vegetables and nourish those frazzled nerves. Thyme can provide feelings of wellbeing. Try bathing with a thyme-infused soap or sip a cup of thyme tea. While you may not be whisked away to an outdoor utopia, these herbs can get you out of your discomfort zone.

DIY CURE #17: FOOT PAIN?
RUN TO LAVENDER AND THYME

Ah, foot pain. This ailment is not uncommon. There are DIY treatments you can try. If you are on your feet working or exercising all day and overdo it, your feet may ache. Or if you wear poor-fitting shoes it can aggravate a bunion or hammertoes. Believe it or not, you can survive the pain and lessen the throbbing, swollen tootsies, and feel better without seeing a doctor.

What Herbal Rx to Use: In a pan of hot water add 2 teaspoons of your favorite combination of dried herbs (I like lavender and thyme), the ones that have anti-inflammatory compounds. Soak for 10 to 15 minutes.

Why Spicing It Up Works: If your feet are red and swollen or a bunion or callus throbs, it's time to take action. Both lavender and thyme contain anti-inflammatory properties that can soothe throbbing and redness. The end result: Foot pain is relieved as swelling subsides.

DIY CURE #18: GOT GINGIVITIS? RINSE IT WITH CUMIN

Welcome to the world of irritated and inflamed gums called gingivitis. Some common causes of red gums are slacking off on toothbrushing and flossing, coping with stressful events, hormones going haywire, or even genetics. If caught early on you can reverse gingivitis, but if you let it go it can turn into periodontal disease. But there is a spice that can help you to get off the wrong path and clear up irritated gums.

What Herbal Rx to Use: Put a dash of cumin into an 8-ounce cup of chamomile or green tea. After drinking the herbal brew, rinse with warm salt water. Repeat twice daily.

Why Spicing It Up Works: Cumin contains anti-inflammatory compounds as does chamomile. Together these two can work synergistically and lessen inflammation. Also, if you get back on track with a good oral hygiene program, visit your dentist regularly, eat less sugar and more nutrient-dense whole foods, you can beat plaque and tartar and enjoy healthy gums and be pain-free.

DIY CURE #19: SENSING GOUT PAIN?
KICK IT WITH FENNEL

Ever hear of gout, a type of arthritis that happens when the body accumulates crystallization of uric acid in your joints? When gout occurs, more often in men, it causes pain in certain joints, which can affect knees, feet, and even the big toe.

What Herbal Rx to Use: Chew 1 teaspoon of fennel seeds or heat an 8-ounce cup of water. Add 1 teaspoon fennel seeds and steep for 3 minutes. Drain. Drink the fennel tea. Repeat daily.

Why Spicing It Up Works: Fennel acts as a diuretic and may get rid of uric acid crystals, the culprits that can create joint pain. There is no hard-hitting proof to claim fennel is the answer to curing a gout flare-up. Still, fennel can help guard you against gout, especially if you add it to a Mediterranean diet, complete with fruits, vegetables, and whole grains. Also, losing unwanted pounds is also advised for an anti-gout lifestyle.

DIY CURE #20: HEADACHE AGONY?
CAYENNE PEPPER TO HALT

Headaches come in all varieties, including cluster, tension, and migraine. Taking an over-the-counter pain reliever often works. But there is an all-natural remedy, thanks to cayenne pepper, that works, too.

What Herbal Rx to Use: Try dabbing a small amount of capsaicin cream inside your nostrils. Use sparingly.

Why Spicing It Up Works: In the chapter on cayenne, I note its ingredient capsaicin and how it works to beat pain. Headaches can be painful. A topical cream method has been used in studies on migraine sufferers and the outcome is pain relief. How? How does it work? Scientists claim capsaicin interrupts pain messengers to the brain. It's worth a try. But note, there can be some burning with the cream.[2]

DIY Cure #21: Heartburn Pain? Fennel Kills It

An occasional bout of heartburn can hit at any time and be uncomfortable. The causes can vary, including acidic food like tomato sauce, onions, and too much garlic. Also, overeating, and eating too fast when emotionally upset, can cause acid reflex. There's good news: When it comes to heartburn, fennel can often be your herbal remedy solution for fast relief.

What Herbal Rx to Use: Brew 1 cup of hot water. Add 1 teaspoon roasted fennel seeds. Steep for 2 to 3 minutes. Strain. Drink as need up to 2 times per day. Or simply chew 1 teaspoon fennel seeds.

Why Spicing It Up Works: Fennel is an ancient remedy for digestive complaints, including acid reflex. It is believed its compound anethole helps to calm the digestive tract. These days, I rarely suffer from heartburn. Occasionally, though, overindulging in hot, spicy food with onions, like salsa, can cause the scourge of heartburn. A neighbor of mine was visiting me during the holidays. One afternoon after admitting to overindulging the night before in wine and rich food, I brewed a cup of fennel tea. It worked!

DIY Cure #22: Irksome Insomnia? Get Shut-Eye with Fennel

Sleepless nights are an unwelcome visitor. Often it can be due to a busy mind, worrying about life stressors, which can be positive. Taking a test, going on a trip, relocating can all be things that keep us tossing and turning. Personally, I hear clock chimes: 1 chime for 1:00 A.M., 2 chimes for 2:00 A.M. But if you're finding it difficult to fall asleep, there is an herb that may do the trick.

What Herbal Rx to Use: Put 1 teaspoon loose fennel seeds or a store-bought tea bag into an 8-ounce to 10-ounce cup of hot water. Steep for 5 minutes. Add honey or milk. Sip and savor the sleepy time herbal tea.

Why Spicing It Up Works: Folklore remedy enthusiasts will tell you fennel works for insomnia, but they don't tell you how it does the job.

Studies published in scientific journals pinpoint all of the mighty components in fennel and L-tryptophan, also found in foods like bananas and turkey, are key ingredients that may be the answer to sweet dreams. It is used to counter insomnia, anxiety, and depression. Simply put, the body uses tryptophan, an amino acid, to make serotonin and melatonin, two mood and sleep-regulating brain messengers in your brain.

One pre-dawn I couldn't sleep because of howling wind before a forecasted snowstorm. My calming chamomile tea box of tea bags was empty. Then, I remembered fennel tea may be the trick to fight my Sleepless in Tahoe night. One large cup of the licorice-like aroma brew, I fell asleep in between the cuddly cat and fluffy dog as the fire in the fireplace dimmed out into embers.

Getting Sound Sleep with an Herbal Cocktail

Medical doctors will tell you anxiety, hormones, stress, indigestion, pain, and even some medications can all trigger occasional sleepless nights and broken sleep. For insomnia, herbs such as these nature's sedatives mixed with good bedtime habits may help you get to sleep.

For shut-eye herbal relief, measure ½ cup chamomile flowers, 1 teaspoon lavender flowers, 1 teaspoon sage leaves, and 1 teaspoon thyme leaves. Combine herbs. Take a teaspoon of the herb mixture and add to 1 cup of hot water. Let sit for 3 minutes. Strain. Add honey to taste. Sip before bedtime.

DIY CURE #23: IRRITABLE BOWEL SYNDROME? CARDAMOM CAN HELP

Life would be perfect if we all would go to the bathroom like clockwork every morning. But reality is imperfect and sometimes factors get in the way of bowel movements. Stress, weather changes, travel are some culprits that can get you off track of being regular. Worse, you can have days without going to the bathroom and then BAM! You can't seem to get off (or on) the toilet. While anise can work, there are other herbal remedies, too.

What Herbal Rx to Use: Remove the shell of 1 cardamom pod. Crush the pod into powder. Brew an 8-ounce cup of water infused with 1 peppermint tea bag. Stir in powder. Add honey to taste. Drink 1 to 2 cups daily.

Why Spicing It Up Works: Cardamom contains the compound cineole, an anti-inflammatory. Combined with peppermint the two herbs can help calm and prevent gas and bloat, two symptoms of IBS. It may help to lessen the discomfort of irregularity. Case-in-point: My friend, a thirty-two-year-old woman, was suffering from IBS. As a goal-oriented Realtor, medical lab technician, and mom of two girls, she often was stressed out. Before showing a home, she would get an IBS flare-up. I suggested the cardamom-peppermint tea cure. The next time I saw her she was more relaxed and energetic. She gave credit to the "magical" tea drink.

DIY Cure #24: Joint Stiffness?
Limber Up with Turmeric

Stiff joints in your legs, arms, and back isn't just a problem for your grandparents. It can happen to anyone at any age (even you!) for many reasons, including a sports injury or a car accident or even being too sedentary. Exercising on a regular basis can keep the body limber. So, what to do if you discover one day that you're walking like a robot in slow motion? Turn to one spice that can also be beneficial to keep your joints useful without pain.

What Herbal Rx to Use: Include turmeric in your diet. It can be consumed in soups, the main course of a meal to beverages. You can also take a supplement.

Why Spicing It Up Works: Turmeric contains curcumin, a phytochemical that can lessen inflammation. Ever notice if your knees or one arm to one finger are stiff? Sure, it's easy to take an over-the-counter anti-inflammatory pill. But turning to the yellow-colored powder turmeric is a spice to write about.

Some scientific studies show that the key compound curcumin may prevent joint inflammation and stiffness linked to rheumatoid arthritis and osteoarthritis. It is also believed turmeric blocks inflammatory cytokine and enzymes. That means you will have bolstered your joint health against the causes that can bring on a bout of joint stiffness.

DIY CURE #25: LOW LIBIDO? GET CLOSE TO CARDAMOM

Inhibited sexual desire can affect both women and men. The cause is multi-faceted. A low libido can be ignited by either physical or psychological reasons. Age, hormones, medications, intimacy issues can play a role in saying, "Not tonight. I have a headache." If it's not an ongoing problem or not due to an underlying health cause, turn to herbs for a little help. An herbal remedy may be just what you need to rev up that loving feeling and enjoy the thrill of intimacy.

What Herbal Rx to Use: Try making strong coffee or tea, with this recipe from Mountain Rose Herbs. Use 1½ teaspoons whole cardamom seeds with 2½ ounces coffee beans. Add 1½ cups water and brew. You can use a few pods, ground, or a dash of ground cardamom in hot chocolate, too.

Why Spicing It Up Works: A cardamom-infused beverage may enhance your sex drive. Or not. It's believed to have aphrodisiac qualities. It could be that the spice helps boost blood circulation, which can work for both men and women in the sex department. No hard-hitting studies prove that it is a natural "love drug," but herbal folklore suggests it may work wonders. If it doesn't work, the caffeine in the cardamom spicy beverage will give you an energizing buzz and the drive to engage in lovemaking, and we know sex can increase endorphins.

DIY CURE #26: MEMORY PAUSES?
REMEMBER SAFFRON

We all have experienced memory lapses, whether it be forgetting a person's name or a character in a movie. It's an unsettling moment when you can't recall where you parked your car or remember a phone number you have memorized. There are spices that can help you to keep your memory sharp. (Oops I forgot which one. Just kidding.) Enter saffron.

What Herbal Rx to Use: Include saffron by either adding it to your seafood (a brain food), rice, and even desserts.

Why Spicing It Up Works: Saffron contains the compound crocin. It is believed by some researchers that it can stall cognitive decline. Past studies suggest crocin can enhance comprehension and help to retain memory. Pair saffron with antioxidant-rich vegetables to get rid of damaging free radicals. Try antioxidant supplements, too, to enhance brain cell energy. I experienced my beloved dog affected by cognitive canine decline (he was twelve and a half years old), and a friend of mine is in a drug trial study that may prevent Alzheimer's. I continue to call myself "elephant" because the saying, "An elephant never forgets." But for extra precaution, I have been including a bit of saffron in my Mediterranean diet.

DIY CURE #27: NERVOUS TENSION?
CHILLAX WITH NUTMEG

If your mind is racing about stressful situations, such as your job, a relationship, or money matters, your thoughts can take a toll on your nervous system. If you can't chill, are on edge, not focused, and irritated easily, it is time to calm your frazzled nerves.

What Herbal Rx to Use: Try using chamomile (1 tea bag or 1 teaspoon loose leaf) brewed as an 8-ounce cup of tea with a small amount of nutmeg. Use once daily.

Why Spicing It Up Works: Researchers point to the compounds in nutmeg that work as a muscle relaxant to help lessen nervousness. When your mind and body are calm, the fight-or-flight stress response is less and a sense of balance happens. Nervous tension can affect your muscles so they feel tight. Ever notice when you get a massage that you feel all wound up? After tension-reducing techniques are used you feel relaxed, right? Nutmeg can be nature's remedy to substitute for a personal masseuse.

Shake the Winter Blues, the Herbal-ish Way!

During late autumn and through winter months, many of us fall victim to the winter doldrums. Shorter days, longer nights, and less sunshine can wreak havoc on the body and mind. When planning the trip to Anchorage (third attempt), I discovered during winter months there are about five or six hours of daylight. So, what to do? What herbs and spices can help you uplift your spirit while surviving Old Man Winter? Here, take a look at herbalism and how it can take care of you to weather colder seasons and stay well.

Vitamin D: Parsley contains vitamin D, the sunshine must-have vitamin (also available in fortified juice and milk and supplements) to include in your daily regime.

Get Moving: Some herbs and spices contain components that can boost physical energy. The energizing spices include cayenne.

Boost Mood: Not unlike vitamin D and energizing herbs and spices, there are seasonings that can uplift your spirit like using happy light box therapy. Anise and cayenne are mood enhancers, happy spices.

DIY CURE #28: MUCUS CYST? GO TO TURMERIC

A small bump inside the mouth, often near the palate or cheek, can be a benign cyst filled with mucus. It is usually painless and a couple of millimeters in size. You can feel it with the tip of your tongue or finger. Simply put, it is a blocked salivary gland. It can be due to postnasal drip, stress, not drinking enough water, or even some medications.

What Herbal Rx to Use: Combine a dash of turmeric powder with ½ teaspoon raw honey. Mix the two ingredients to form a paste. Dab it on the cyst. Rinse after 15 minutes. Use this remedy 2 or 3 times per day.

Why Spicing It Up Works: Turmeric contains curcumin. Not only is the yellow powder a good anti-inflammatory, but it also is a good natural antibacterial agent. A mucus cyst usually will go away within a few days. During one dental check-up, I asked my dentist about the tiny lump. Without hesitation, he explained to me that it was a blocked gland. I blamed the cyst on my allergies and sinusitis, which can cause pesky mucus buildup in the throat. I tried this turmeric remedy and drank more water and tea. The cyst was gone within one day.

DIY CURE #29: HELLO, NAUSEA?
SAY GOOD-BYE WITH CLOVE

Nobody enjoys feeling nauseous or queasy, which can happen for a number of reasons. Morning sickness, a stressful event, motion sickness, an inner ear issue from flushing earwax with water that is too cold, or going on an amusement park ride. All of these up-and-down roller-coaster-type events we cannot control can be met with that telltale time that you may be sick to your stomach. But sometimes with a folk remedy you can stave off that uneasy, queasy visitor and feel normal again.

What Herbal Rx to Use: Brew a cup of hot water. Add 1 clove, crushed. Stir until blended. Or chew on 1 clove.

Why Spicing It Up Works: Sipping a cup of fragrant clove tea can soothe your tummy. Cloves contain eugenol, which provides antibacterial properties. The soothing aroma can help stave off that telltale queasy feeling you get before being sick. Also, cloves can help speed the digestion process and lessen cramps that sometimes accompany nausea. I purchase a black tea with sweet orange and clove. The autumn blend is pleasant, and orange can also soothe an upset stomach.

DIY CURE #30: PMS CRAMPS? TRICK IT WITH FENNEL

Women in childbearing years can experience the scourge of premenstrual syndrome, and that includes cramps. Cramps in the pelvic region can be minimal to even debilitating where it's almost a must to cozy up with a heating pad to relieve the constant pain. There is an herbal remedy that can help ease the throbbing, dull pain. Enter a soothing wonder that may provide relief.

What Seasoning Rx to Use: Heat 1 cup of water. Add 1 teaspoon dried fennel seeds. Steep for 3 minutes. Strain. Add honey to taste. Repeat as needed. Also, chewing 1 teaspoon of fennel seeds can work.

Why Spicing It Up Works: I can personally attest to surviving PMS throughout my twenties and into menopause. I took an over-the-counter medication Midol, but it had side effects with its caffeine, and didn't help the pre-menstrual crankies where you want to be alone. Fennel contains the antispasmodic anethole (a compound to soothe spasms) that may help to lessen menstrual cramps in women. Iran researchers conducted a study where sixty young women were given drops of fennel. The herb did help quell cramps but complaints of the unpleasant taste were reported.[3]

DIY CURE #31: POSTMENOPAUSAL HAVOC? MORE FENNEL

Welcome to menopause—during and after one year without a period. Symptoms can last a decade. Worse, post-menopause hot flashes, sleeplessness, and vaginal dryness can be nightmare-ish. A baby boomer friend of mine shared her misery of experiencing hot flashes at night during her tossing and turning during sleepless nights. She was frustrated and didn't know what to do or take. Medical researchers get credit for their studies on how herbal medicine can be effective to reduce post-menopause demons.

What Herbal Rx to Use: Try an 8-ounce cup of hot water with 1 organic fennel tea bag. Repeat twice daily as needed.

Why Spicing It Up Works: Fennel, an anise-flavored culinary herb, can help lessen hot flashes, sleeplessness, vaginal dryness, and anxiety without troublesome side effects of hormone therapy. Iran researchers found fennel contains phytoestrogen, an estrogen-like chemical in plants, can treat menopause symptoms. Their findings were published in *Menopause*, the journal of the North American Menopause Society. In a small study of seventy-nine Iranian middle-aged women, soft capsules containing 100 milligrams of fennel were given twice daily for two months. The fennel supplement improved menopause symptoms, but a larger study is still needed to announce definitive proof it works.[4]

DIY CURE #32: GOT PSORIASIS?
FIND RELIEF WITH CAYENNE

Welcome to psoriasis, a chronic condition where skin cells multiply too fast and build up. This, in turn, results in scaly, red, and irritated patches. These blotches can show up on the scalp, elbows, palms, knees, and soles of the feet.

What Herbal Rx to Use: Try using over-the-counter products containing capsaicin. Follow directions and apply the topical remedy for relief and healing.

Spicing It Up Works: Capsaicin, the main compound in cayenne, may help heal scaly skin, redness, and itching. It helps to lessen inflammation, which is the culprit for the scourge of this ailment. In the twentieth century, a friend of mine told me about her cousin who suffered from the physical and emotional pain of psoriasis. It was an unwelcome visitor that affected her well-being, especially with her husband. The skin condition caused her to feel inhibited and uncomfortable during lovemaking. I remember saying, "There must be some type of treatment to aid her skin." But the woman let each flare-up run its course and was miserable.

DIY CURE #33: RECEDING GUMS?
TIGHTEN UP WITH CLOVE

Imagine the ocean and its ebb and flow. Well, unfortunately as we age our gums can recede like the ocean. Other causes can be poor oral hygiene, excess bacteria and plaque, and even hormones. On the upside, we can slow down receding gums—and one healing spice may help. Also, there is a home remedy for you to try.

What Herbal Rx to Use: Crush 1 clove with 1 teaspoon olive oil. Apply clove paste to your gum. Rinse 10 minutes afterward. Repeat 2 times daily.

Spicing It Up Works: Clove oil is a known remedy for a toothache or gum irritation. But cloves contain antibacterial compounds, too. That means it may help fight minor gum inflammation. Try chewing a clove instead of taking antibiotics or running to a periodontist. Getting your teeth professionally cleaned on a regular basis, using an electric toothbrush, and flossing daily can help slow down recession, too.

DIY CURE #34: ROSACEA REDNESS?
GHOST IT WITH TURMERIC

Ah, rosacea and I go back in time. In a nutshell, rosacea is a skin condition that fair-skinned people often endure. Redness and visible blood vessels in your face show up. Working out, heat, extreme temperature changes, all can be causes and culprits. During grad school oral exams, I was a bundle of nerves, which led me to a dermatologist. He prescribed anti-anxiety medication and a topical anti-inflammatory steroid cream. Also, doctor's orders were to shun the sun.

What Herbal Rx to Use: Sprinkle turmeric ground powder sparingly on top of foods, such as soups and stews. Also, you can try turmeric supplements available online or at the drugstore.

Why Spicing It Up Works: The antioxidant curcumin in turmeric acts as an anti-inflammatory without the side effects of steroids. Caveat: Turmeric may be helpful in lessening the redness, but lifestyle changes, including destressing and staying out of the sun, are part of the anti-rosacea regimen. The upside: If you have rosacea, often you'll be burdened by flare-ups but overall you can control it.

DIY Cure #35: Sore Throat? Sip Turmeric

A sore throat can be caused by many things, including a precursor to a common cold, laryngitis, and allergies. Dr. Anil Minocha, a gastroenterologist based in Surprise, Arizona, touts the "golden" herb powder. "My favorite is turmeric. I use it a lot. Virtually every meal I cook has turmeric," he says. "When I have a cold or sore throat," the doctor adds, "I mix it in lukewarm milk." A turmeric mixture with milk is nothing new, but it is new to me as it may be to you.

What Herbal Rx to Use: Heat 8 ounces of organic 2 percent low-fat milk. Heat it up on the stovetop and bring to a boil and remove. Add ½ teaspoon ground turmeric and a dash of ground black pepper. Let set for 5 minutes. Add raw honey if you prefer a sweet kick. Drink twice daily, ideally once in the morning and repeat at night.

Why Spicing It Up Works: The good doctor knows, as other health experts do, that the Indian spice boasts curcumin, a rich spice with anti-inflammatory benefits. This, in turn, can help reduce redness and swelling of a tender throat. The pepper helps your body to absorb the yellow herb so it will do its job and soothe a sore throat.

DIY Cure #36: Spacey Mind? Focus with Cloves

Feeling distracted, fogged, spaced-out? We've all experienced brain fog or fuzzy concentration at one time or another. It can happen when we're overworked, experiencing a stressful event, jet lag, and desperately need a good night's sleep. Usually, this mindlessness will pass, but you can do something to get mentally energized. This herb can really help boost mental clarity, mood, and ability to focus.

What Herbal Rx to Use: Try crushing up a few cloves. Heat an 8-ounce cup of water to a boil. Steep cloves in the water for 3 to 5 minutes. Add ½ teaspoon to a cup of black tea or coffee.

Why Spicing It Up Works: Cloves are a known mental energizer. Scientists believe its credit goes to eugenol, the antioxidant in cloves known to boost brain chemicals or "neurotransmitters" that enhance both serotonin and dopamine—the feel-good chemical messengers in your brain. This, in result, can clear your mind and help you feel a sense of well-being, and more focused and alert at work or play.

I personally fell in love with a pumpkin spice coffee made with both natural and artificial flavors including cloves and nutmeg. After the first cup my mind was clear and ready to accomplish any mental challenge. The scent of the coffee in the bag and mug were stimulating.

DIY CURE #37: SPIDER BITES AND STINGS: SHOO PAIN WITH PARSLEY

Ever been bit by a spider (or another creepy crawler)? Not only does the initial bite sting it can throb. Living in the mountains for two decades, I've been bitten more than once. One toxic spider bite put me at the clinic on a weekend. A tetanus shot later, I was still in pain. Nothing I used at home offered relief except time and knowing I wouldn't get lockjaw. Later, I discovered there is an herbal remedy that can relieve the sting.

What Herbal Rx to Use: Put 2 tablespoons parsley, fresh or dried, into a pot of hot water. Strain the tea and apply to skin three times per day. Repeat for a few days.

Why Spicing It Up Works: Parsley contains antibacterial and anti-inflammatory compounds. Both of these can stop infection and pain from a swollen bite. A parsley poultice is refreshing, easy to make, and doesn't smell. When I was an outdoorsy-loving child, a bug spray or yucky pink calamine lotion was the twentieth-century remedy to soothe throbbing pain from a bug bite. Instead of using these stinky treatments, it's easier and less costly to heal a spider bite with a parsley tea.

DIY Cure #38: Sprain Pain?
Break Time with Garlic

A sprain is not as bad as breaking a leg or dislocating a kneecap. But when you sprain your wrist or ankle, it hurts. After the damage is done, inflammation kicks in and throbbing and discomfort follow. A doctor will tell you that RICE (rest, ice, compress, and elevation) can help heal a sprain. And, of course, time heals. So, in a rush so you can use that body part?

What Herbal Rx to Use: Mince ½ cup fresh garlic and put it into a glass container. Pour olive oil over the herb. Let it rest in a warm area for a few days. Once you have homemade garlic oil, smooth it on the sprained region. Repeat a few times per day.

Why Spicing It Up Works: The anti-inflammatory compounds in garlic oil (and olive oil) can help lessen swelling and redness. One time I accidentally bent back my middle finger. It hurt so bad that I went to bed that night. In the morning my finger was swollen and bruised. I went to the doctor and was given a splint. It was not broken or fractured. The glitch is, I was on deadline to submit a hundred pages to a college as part of being accepted into the graduate program. The day after the mishap, I took off the splint and massaged my finger with garlic oil. Then, I continued to crank out the words on the typewriter. Did it hurt? Yes. But did my finger heal? Yes, and I was accepted into the program. I give credit to the garlic oil treatment.

DIY Cure #39: Stressed-Out?
Lighten Up with Marjoram

Life comes with a mixed bag of daily stressors. You, like me, likely face stressors, from time to time, which can be due to issues about family, work, money, health, or the fish that went belly-up. Stress can be combined with anxiety and depression. There are herbs to help you to stay chill, especially used with an arsenal of Mediterranean-plant-based diet and lifestyle changes.

What Herbal Rx to Use: Heat 12 ounces of hot water. Add ½ teaspoon of each dried marjoram and oregano to the water and steep for 3 minutes. Strain and drink the herbal tea. Repeat twice daily as needed.

Why Spicing It Up Works: Both stress-relieving herbs can help calm your nervous system due to antispasmodic compounds that work to soothe digestive distress and muscular spasms. When you're tense your body can feel tight. These two anti-stress herbs help to relax the body and mind. And finding your om mantra can't hurt.

DIY CURE #40: TENDINITIS PAIN?
GET RELIEF WITH CAYENNE

Tendons at any age can become stiff and sore. Often it is caused by repetitive movement like at work or play. When joints are swollen and inflamed it can hurt and your arms or legs will be stiff. A doctor will prescribe an anti-steroid cream to lessen inflammation. But the first remedy that may give you relief is an herb.

What Herbal Rx to Use: Use an over-the-counter cream with capsaicin (a compound in cayenne) on the tender region. Repeat as needed and follow the instructions.

Why Spicing It Up Works: The first time I discovered the pain benefits of cayenne was when I was assigned a health article on natural remedies for pain. One of the top cures was cayenne. I discussed its power was due to the anti-inflammatory compounds in capsaicin. One summer years later, my sibling complained of a sore hand. He connected the pain to his regular game of golf. He was ready to try CBD oil because of its popularity. I suggested the cayenne treatment since it has a long history of beating pain. After resistance he took my advice. I didn't hear any more complaints.

DIY CURE #41: TONSILLITIS SORENESS?
FIND COMFORT WITH GARLIC

Often youngsters will have their tonsils surgically removed at an early age, as I did at two. But some kids don't have problems until later. My older sister didn't have the procedure until she was eight. After the hospital stay, healing took time. At after-school daycare one afternoon, I recall watching her trying to eat a sandwich at the kitchen table. But observing her conceal pieces of food into a napkin showed me it hurt her to swallow. In hindsight, I wonder why the caretaker didn't provide popsicles—or a home remedy to soothe the pain.

What Herbal Rx to Use: In a saucepan, bring to a boil 3 minced cloves of garlic in 2 cups of water. Add 2 tablespoons lemon juice and 2 table-spoons honey. Take 2 tablespoons of the garlic syrup 3 times per day.

Why Spicing It Up Works: Garlic has both antibacterial and anti-viral compounds. Crushing garlic before usage boosts its allicin content. Combining the herb with honey (especially for a child) makes it more mildly seasoned. Both garlic and honey can lessen the redness and swelling of a sore throat. Also, lemon and honey contain antioxidants that bolster the immune system to fight inflammation and can soothe pain in the throat when swallowing. While I didn't remember my op-eration, I do recall having strep throat so I could empathize with the hurt.

DIY Cure #42: Toothache Throbbing? Chew a Clove

Can you stop the big throb with little cloves? Maybe. An aching tooth can affect people of all ages—a cavity or leaky filling can hurt or a chipped tooth. Often a dental emergency seems to happen at night, holiday, or on vacation when a dentist is AWOL. When I bit into a dried fig, I broke an upper molar. Clove oil was my best friend for a weekend out of town until a dental appointment.

What Herbal Rx to Use: Crush up 1 clove into a powder. Mix it with a bit of olive oil until you have a paste. Dab it on the aching tooth. Repeat as necessary.

Why Spicing It Up Works: One late Friday afternoon I was chewing on a dried fig. I felt and heard a loud "crunch" in my mouth. I took out a piece of the chewy fruit and a tiny piece of my upper back molar greeted me. Immediately I called my dentist. Since he was gone until Monday and I was scheduled to go out of town—pain medication was the doctor's orders. If I could replay that weekend, I would have tried cloves. It is the compound eugenol in cloves and clove essential oil that can quickly numb the pain. It is a quick fix. Cloves will not heal a chipped tooth but it may stop the throbbing until the tooth is taken care of by the dentist. (Epilogue: I did save the tooth with a crown. And I vowed to give up dried figs for eternity.)

DIY Cure #43: Urinary Tract Infection? Go Find Garlic

A urinary tract infection (UTI) is when the bladder swells, gets irritated, and is inflamed. The cause is due to bacteria, usually E. coli. It can be due to sex, hormonal changes, thanks to declining estrogen after menopause, and even a polluted hot tub or pool. Symptoms include an urgency to urinate, burning, and even pelvic pain. If it is a mild bladder infection it can go away on its own within a few days. But there are ways to speed up the healing process with nature's cure— garlic.

What Herbal Rx to Use: Eat ½ garlic clove, raw and minced. It's best to spread it with olive oil on a piece of toasted bread. Or try garlic tea available online. Drink a 12-ounce glass of water after ingesting garlic. Repeat twice a day.

Why Spicing It Up Works: Garlic contains allicin, which works as an anti-inflammatory and antibacterial compound. Once the urgency to urinate stops, inflammation is less and pain goes way. A UTI can be cured at home (often without a doctor's prescription for a drug that comes with side effects). Note: If you feel an infection coming on, as a preventive measure drink cranberry juice once daily. Always drink 6 to 8 (8-ounce) glasses of water daily. And, add garlic to your diet.

HEALING HIGHLIGHTS FROM NATURE'S GARDEN-FEST

If it doesn't explain the method of herb or spice to use, follow your judgment and personal preference. For instance, if you do not like to eat garlic you can try a garlic supplement. Or if you would rather sip parsley tea than nibble on a parsley sprig—no worries. It's all good.

Ailment	Herb/Spice	What It Can Do
✓ Anxiety	Allspice	Relaxes nervous system
✓ Bad breath	Parsley	Rids of odor
✓ Bloating	Dill	Rids of water weight
✓ Blood clots	Garlic	Thins blood, enhances circulation
✓ Bruises	Parsley	Heals discolored skin, swelling
✓ Cold	Garlic	Guards against bacteria
✓ Congestion	Cayenne	Opens nasal passages, dries postnasal drip
✓ Conjunctivitis	Cilantro	Soothes irritation
✓ Constipation	Fennel	Boosts regularity
✓ Cough	Cardamom	Stops irritation, tickle
✓ Cuts, punctures	Garlic	Fights bacteria, swelling
✓ Earache	Turmeric	Lessens pain, inflammation
✓ Fever	Cilantro	Detoxifies, enhances immune system
✓ Fibromyalgia	Cayenne	Relieves aches and pains
✓ Flatulence	Fennel	Lessens gas, discomfort

Ailment	Herb/Spice	What It Can Do
✓ Foot pain	Lavender, thyme	Relieves swelling, pain
✓ Flu	Cayenne cocktail	Bolsters immunity
✓ Gingivitis	Cumin	Lessens irritation, redness
✓ Gout	Fennel	Rids crystals
✓ Headache	Cayenne	Beats pain, tightness
✓ Heartburn	Fennel	Aids in digestion, calms
✓ Insomnia	Fennel	Boosts melatonin to calm
✓ Irritable Bowel Syndrome	Cardamom	Aids digestion, mind
✓ Joint stiffness	Turmeric	Lessens tightness
✓ Low libido	Cardamom	Boosts blood circulation
✓ Memory pauses	Saffron	Enhances brain cells
✓ Nervous tension	Nutmeg	Relaxes nervous system
✓ Mucus cyst	Turmeric	Unblocks swollen gland
✓ Nausea	Clove	Soothes stomach
✓ PMS cramps, crankies	Fennel	Calms spasms, pain
✓ Postmenopausal woes	Fennel	Eases symptoms naturally
✓ Psoriasis	Cayenne	Lessens itching, redness
✓ Receding gums	Clove	Relieves swollen tissue
✓ Rosacea	Turmeric	Rids of redness
✓ Sore throat	Turmeric	Calms burn, tenderness

Ailment	Herb/Spice	What It Can Do
✓ Spacy mind	Clove	Boost brain clarity
✓ Spider bites, stings	Parsley	Calms pain, swelling
✓ Sprain	Garlic	Lessens pain, swelling
✓ Stress	Marjoram, Cilantro	Relaxes nervous system
✓ Tendinitis	Cayenne	Relieves swelling tightness
✓ Tonsillitis	Garlic	Fights redness, pain
✓ Toothache	Clove	Numbs throbbing
✓ Urinary tract	Garlic	Fights inflammation, pain

From Gourmet Garden Herbs & Spices
(used with permission)

HERB OR SPICE	POTENTIAL HEALTH BENEFITS
Garlic	Antioxidant, lowers cholesterol and blood pressure, raises HDL cholesterol, anti-inflammatory, prevents cerebral aging, anti-clotting, boosts immunity
Ginger	Antioxidant, improves osteoarthritis of the knee, anti-emetic, anti-inflammatory, boosts immunity, antimicrobial
Lemon Grass	Antioxidant, anti-cancer properties, anti-inflammatory
Cilantro	Antioxidant, digestive aid
Chili	Antioxidant, enhances metabolic effects in weight management
Basil	Antioxidant, inhibits lipid peroxidation, decreases inflammation
Dill	Antioxidant, antimicrobial
Parsley	Antioxidant, antimicrobial
Oregano	Antioxidant, antimicrobial
Marjoram	Antioxidant, antimicrobial
Thyme	Antioxidant, inhibits bone resorption
Rosemary	Antioxidant, inhibits bone resorption, anti-carcinogen, anti-inflammatory

SUGGESTED USES

World cuisine, meat, seafood, poultry, stir-fry: use in marinades, dressings, sauces, salads, rice dishes and casseroles; also use in slow-cooked meals and as a rub for meats, toppings (bruschetta) and dips, vegetables, beans, tofu.

Asian style cuisine, meat, seafood, poultry, stir-fry, curries: use in marinades, chutneys and desserts; also use to flavor fruit smoothies and tea, soups, vegetables, cocoa, fruits.

Asian style cuisine, seafood, shrimp, poultry and stir-fry; also use in soups, curries and rice dishes and noodles, tofu and custards.

Asian, Middle Eastern, Latin and Mexican style cuisine: use in cooked dishes, dressings, dipping sauces, salads, soups, marinades and rubs as well as shellfish.

Asian, Mediterranean, African and Latin inspired cuisine, meat, poultry, seafood: use in marinades, dipping sauces and curries, soups and stews, pasta sauces, rice and egg dishes.

Mediterranean or Asian style cuisine: use with tomatoes or as a base for pesto, in salads, sauces, marinades, as a drizzle for soups and vegetables and cooked dishes.

Mediterranean and American style cuisine: use with seafood, dipping sauces, potato salads, vegetables, chicken, soups and marinades.

World cuisine: use with potato or pasta salads; also use raw or cooked with meats, vegetables, shellfish and seafood.

Mediterranean style cuisine, meat, fish, poultry: use with vegetables, breads, salad dressing, pasta, sauces and marinades.

Mediterranean, African, Middle Eastern and American cuisines: use with meat, fish, poultry, vegetables, breads, salad dressings and stuffings.

Mediterranean style cuisine: use in soups, casseroles, stuffings, salad dressings and marinades, rubs & vegetables.

Mediterranean style cuisine, meat, fish, poultry: use with vegetables, breads, salad dressings, sauces, fall fruits and rice dishes.

PART 5

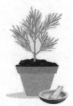

SHAKING IT UP

Beauty and the Season(ings)

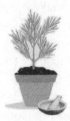

*Is not birth, beauty, good shaper, discourse, manhood,
learning, Gentleness, virtue, youth, liberality, and
such like, the spice and salt that season a man.*
—WILLIAM SHAKESPEARE, *Scene II The Same. A street.*

En route solo to Toronto, Canada, I was in dire need of self-pampering
and beautifying me time from head to toe. It was a long trek from Lake
Tahoe to Eastern Canada. I destressed in a soaker tub. I used my own
combination of store-bought herbs (lavender and thyme) in a facial
and hair conditioner. An exfoliant for my body was just what I needed
after a day of travel. The oversized tub overlooking Lake Ontario in
the spring and the city skyline with the aroma of herbs (I brought tea
bags to chill) rejuvenated me. I created my own personal spa night.
And on the high hotel floor suite I was in herbal heaven.

Luxury spas at resort hotels, destination health resorts, hair salons,
and skin clinics around the globe offer ancient herbs and spices in
their cutting-edge beauty treatments. A typical spa menu may include

herbal facials, massages, baths, body wraps, pedicures, and more. Spice blends, such as pumpkin spice, are big, and spice and herb blends are used at luxury day spas and spa resorts.

For decades spas have been offering herbal treatments, but these days not only do spas grow their own herbs on the premises but some allow their guests to go outdoors to the resort's garden to pick herbs to be used in their treatments. Other spa resorts make it easier, and roll in a cart full of herbs into the treatment room.

It's bringing nature to guests and its fresh herbs and the ability to choose the aromatic ones that make it a personalized, custom-tailored spa experience. Spa therapists will tell you it's fun for guests to choose different herbs, including chamomile to lavender, so they can enjoy the aroma and healing powers just for their needs.

Some posh hotels, such as the Ritz-Carlton San Francisco, use a Mediterranean flower called immortal in one of their beauty treatments. Los Angeles offers a rooftop garden, like I've seen in Hallmark films on TV. Both spas use garden gifts for scrubs, masques, wraps, and baths.

Other resorts in the United States and in exotic countries are found on farms. The spa sources their herbs for beauty treatments. The Pumpkin Spice Body Wrap being one in demand, especially during autumn and holiday season. Not to forget other spas have large greenhouses that are a source of Mediterranean herbs, such as parsley and thyme. Herbs are organic and seasonal. Guests can chill in the outdoor garden and even cut an herb of choice to use in their spa treatment or beverage.

Here, take a look at herbal treatments paired with fragrant herbs that have been used by royalty centuries ago.

Aromatherapy Massage: With this herbal treatment, you get a massage with aromatic essential oils that are extracted from herbs. Often, guests will choose herbs, such as lavender, to help calm the nervous system.

European Facial: These deep-cleansing treatments include a gentle, exfoliating peel, a massage, and a nourishing mask to rejuvenate your skin. A hydrating hand treatment usually finishes the service. A forty-ish Swedish friend of mine had this treatment done at a day spa. Afterward, her fair skin appeared radiant and glowing. The treatment made her look rested and energized.

There are readymade products online and at spas. I found a honey and saffron facial scrub glow. It promises to exfoliate and cleanse the skin without dehydrating it (a good thing because the air where I live is dry). Also, the product information points out saffron extract lightens skin to reveal more of a glow. Good to know. Note to self: I will give it a go.

Herbal Body Wrap: If you're wondering, "What is a body wrap?" you're not alone. I learned it is a gentle type of body sloughing. Its purpose is to moisturize and detox the skin. Active ingredients also dissolve dead skin cells, making wraps a good exfoliant. Herbal wraps use strips of cloth that have been soaked in herbs and are used to wrap the body. Not only can this beauty treatment smooth the skin, it can lessen the appearance of cellulite, especially if you choose the right herb.

Herbal Treatments at Cal-a-Vie

In Southern California lies a popular health spa called Cal-a-Vie. Not only do they grow herbs on their property, but they use them for beauty treatments. This posh and breathtaking Mediterranean-type spa offers everything to pamper one from head to toe and that includes plant therapy. Seasonal spa treatments are in demand, and this spa with its own garden offers a variety of herbs and spices in their assortment of treatments.

For winter, there is the Peak Purification Body Wrap, which incorporates sage and lavender. Springtime offers a Sol Gemstone Wrap with orange blossoms and black pepper. In summer it's time for Himalayan Super Fruit Body Wrap, which can be enhanced by sipping an herbal iced tea. Last but not to be forgotten is autumn with its Pumpkin Spice Body Wrap.

I interviewed the spa folks to find out more about what herbs they put to work. Take a look at the five questions and answers about herbal bliss—the popular lavender herb is the key player.

Q: *Describe your Herbal Poultice Massage.*

A: With a combination of Swedish massage strokes, gentle pressure, and therapeutic stretching, this unique massage uses Himalayan salt crystals, combined with lavender flowers to restore the body's natural balance and state of well-being. After fifty to ninety minutes, the skin is left feeling softly renewed and nourished.

Q: *What else does the Herbal Poultice Massage do from a health perspective?*

A: It is a relaxing treatment. It is detoxifying by aiding in increased oxygenation of the blood circulation. It aids in inflammation reduction within the joints and muscles. It also remineralizes the skin with the combination of lavender and salt crystals merged with heat.

Q: *Who loves this treatment?*

A: The soothing fragrances of lavender flowers and sea salts appeal to all age groups and genders.

Q: *Ah, speaking of lavender flowers, please describe the Lavender Honey Wrap offered on your spa menu. I enjoyed a honey Jacuzzi bath once and it was true splendor in the herbs. Does this treatment include real herbs?*

A: It uses both the herbs and oils. We also feature our property-harvested honey from our hives. The treatment is ninety minutes and is incredibly relaxing. The wrap begins with a luxurious scrub to exfoliate the skin and improve circulation. Next, warmed honey will be drizzled on your body before you are cocooned in a warming blanket to indulge in the luscious goodness of this wrap. After showering you will receive an application of a lavender-infused lotion.

Q: *Do you recall a guest who benefited from one of these herbal treatments?*

A: It is wonderful to see our guests who are a bit sore from their workouts in the mornings come and enjoy our Herbal Poultice Massage. The best part is that we can target specific areas with this treatment. The warmth of the massage infused with the Himalayan salt and lavender relaxes their muscles and provides herbal relief.

AT-HOME HERBAL BEAUTY

I have treated myself to both a spa herbal bath and manicure. But then it comes to facials I prefer to do it at home. Why? I have sensitive skin and like to be in control of what ingredients I use and how long the facial will last. If you're a bit fussy, like me, there are plenty of facial products available online. Choose your herbs and do it yourself!

Herbal Facial: Want to get your face glow on? Try using a facial scrub gel with honey and saffron. It exfoliates, cleanses the skin without dehydrating it. Saffron extract lightens skin to reveal more of a glowing skin. You can purchase an online product or make it. Mix 4 tablespoons honey with ½ teaspoon saffron powder. Smooth the mixture on your face. Rinse with warm, then cold water after 5 minutes. Blot dry. Follow up with a moisturizer.

Acne Fighter Roll-On: What you'll need: 10 mL roll-on bottle, grapeseed carrier oil, 1 drop oregano essential oil, 2 drops tea tree essential oil. What you'll do: Fill the roll-on bottle with grapeseed carrier oil. Add the essential oils. Apply directly to blemishes 1 to 2 times a day for clear, healthy skin. (Courtesy: Plant Therapy)

Clean Pores: Add 2 thyme or fennel tea bags to 4 cups of hot water and put in a sink or bowl. Cover your head with a towel. Rest your face about 1 foot above the water for about 5 minutes.

Eye Care: To get rid of puffy eyes, wet 2 tea bags (parsley or dandelion) with cool water. Lie down and put a bag over each of your eyelids. Chill for 10 minutes. Remove. Blot eyelids with cold water. Dry.

Tub Soak: Fasten 2 or 3 herbal tea bags (lavender and thyme are nice) under the water faucet when you fill the tub. A bonus tip: Make a cup of chamomile tea to get a double relaxation effect.

Exotic Escapes Bath Salts: What you'll need: 2 tablespoons body wash (your choice), unscented, ½ cup Epsom salt, 2 drops ginger root CO_2 essential oil, 2 drops cardamom essential oil, 1 drop orange sweet essential oil. What you'll do: Mix your body wash and essential oils in a small bowl, and stir. Once the oils and body wash are combined, mix in your Epsom salts. Add to your bath for an exotic scented treat.' (Courtesy: Plant Therapy)

Orange Grove Perfume Rollerball: What you'll need: 10 mL roller bottle, 5 drops sweet orange essential oil, 3 drops neroli essential oil, 1 drop petitgrain essential oil, 1 drop cardamom essential oil, and fractionated coconut oil. What you'll do: In a small bowl, mix your essential oils with fractionated coconut oil. Then pour into your 10 mL roller bottle. Apply to wrists as needed for a fresh scent. (Courtesy: Plant Therapy)

Do note, essential oils are extracted from plants. Essential oils, carrier oils, and roll-on balls to Epsom salts are available online, at aromatherapy and some herbs and spices shops.

Using at-home herbs and spices for beauty is easy and convenient. But sometimes, treating yourself to ready-made products is a pampering treat. Go to your favorite online happy place and search the herbs and spices with the beauty treatment you want. You'll be pleasantly surprised to see all the herbalist beauty products available to you.

**Relaxing and Recharging
Herbal Tub Time Formula**

Fasten 2 to 3 herbal tea bags (chamomile and lavender are nice) under the water faucet when you fill the tub. Also, brew a cup of flavored citrus, clove infused black tea for a rejuvenating effect.

Or for a more homemade cure, try sewing a handful of dried chamomile flowers, dried, crushed bay leaves, and thyme (¼ cup each) into a cheesecloth bag. Hang under a running faucet to infuse a bath. Before you step into the tub—make sure you have a cup of hot herbal tea to sip.

So, you're likely feeling more beautiful on the inside and outside— and now it's time to beautify your home environment, the green way!

HEALING HIGHLIGHTS FROM NATURE'S GARDEN-FEST

✓ You can treat yourself to an herbal treatment at a spa getaway or a day spa. If you choose one service it could be worth the effort, expense, and time.

✓ But note, beauty herbal spa pampering can be done in the comfort of your home, too. Once you get comfortable using different herbs and methods, it's a pleasure you can enjoy more often without breaking the bank.

✓ Before you try a homemade herbal treatment, do use a patch test to ensure that you don't have a reaction to the herb of your choice.

✓ If you enjoy a turmeric beauty treatment, don't forget to treat yourself to a turmeric combo tea (found online or even in grocery stores) for a double effect.

✓ Go ahead—treat yourself to one treatment at a spa or home or make a day of it and pamper yourself from head to toe with nature's herbs and spices.

Flower Power to the
Household

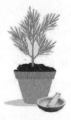

The lovely flowers embarrass me.
They make me regret I am not a bee.
—EMILY DICKINSON

Before I left for a trip to Ontario, Canada, my seventy-three-year-old cabin was cleaned—and I used whole herbs to do the job. While I kenneled the dog, leaving the cat to hold down the fort is one reason why I used nature's cleaners. I filled a jar halfway with sprigs of dried herbs: lavender flowers and thyme—two favorite herbs of springtime. Then, I filled the jar the rest of the way with a half and half mixture of tap water and white vinegar. Not only did it do the work of refreshing the bathroom and kitchen, the fragrance in early spring was wonderful—and it was a memorable aroma that welcomed me when I repeated "There's no place like home." And my Siamese kitty Zen greeted me with purrs, kneading my chest, and cuddling me to sleep after a long journey.

HERBS FOR HOUSE CLEANING

Using fresh or dried herbs for house cleaning is as good at it gets. Some herbs used for an eco-friendly way to freshen up a room and make it dirt-free and tidy include cloves, marjoram, and thyme (from my 22 herbs and spices picks). But other herbs can be used, too, such as cinnamon, citrus peel, lavender, rosemary, and sage.

Herbs can be combined with a variety of solutions. I prefer baking soda for a cleanser scrub because it makes a nice paste mixed with water. White vinegar has antimicrobial and antiseptic properties. A combination of water, vinegar, and lemon juice put in a spray bottle can be used for a variety of clean-up jobs.

Herbs provide antimicrobial, antiseptic, and antifungal properties. If you have used commercial cleaners, you know like I do, they work but the chemical residue smells bad and lingers. Plus, it can affect your nasal membranes and throat if you're sensitive to certain chemicals. It's better to feel good about freshening and cleaning your home with green stuff, rather than the chemical liquids and powders.

INDOORS

Kitchen: In a spray bottle, combine 2 tablespoons thyme, crushed or a couple of sprigs, ¼ cup white vinegar, 1 tablespoon fresh lemon juice, and 1 cup water. This solution can be used to spritz on countertops, inside a microwave, refrigerator, and windows.

Living Room/Dining Room: In a spray bottle, combined ½ cup apple cider vinegar with 2 teaspoons fresh lemon juice and sprigs of fresh lavender. Add 1 cup water. Use a cotton cloth and dust wooden furniture with scratches and smudges. Wipe and buff.

Bedrooms: Add potpourri sachets in drawers of chests and nightstands. Use the seasonal mix for best results.

Bathroom: In a plastic container add ¼ cup baking soda, 2 teaspoons lavender, crushed, and 1 teaspoon lemon juice. Add ½ cup water. Mix well. Use as an abrasive cleanser for the shower or tub, sink, and toilet.

OUTDOORS

Garden Balancer: Marjoram in the garden is beneficial. It's pretty to look at but it works, too! I can attract beautiful butterflies and insects that get rid of pesky pests. This herb, like the hardworking honeybee, can pollinate plants!

Garden Insecticide: Garlic can help guard against unwanted insects. In a pan, combine 15 cloves of garlic in 1 teaspoon mineral oil. Cover. After one day, add ⅛ cup of a natural soap in 8 cups water. Add garlic solution. Strain the mixture and put the garlic liquid into a glass spray bottle. Spritz your garden plants with the spray. Repeat as needed

Wild Edible Flowers

As a Northern California native, I can't help to hum the lyrics, "Be sure to wear some flowers in your hair," a pop song sung by Scott McKenzie, released in May 1967 during the Flower Power hippie era, especially celebrated in San Francisco. But seriously. Can you really eat flowers?

Adding the right edible flowers to dishes as an ingredient or garnish is nothing new. On the Food Network channel some of the chefs, kids and adults, include different flowers on cakes and salad. There is a garden-variety of types of flowers that you can pick and dish up. Try a fresh green salad with herbs and edible garden flowers. Or dish up pumpkin/carrot soup with saffron and edible pansy flowers. Other edible flowers include, dill, fennel, oregano, and tarragon—the herbs from my top 22 herbs and spices collection in this book.

Are edible flowers healthy? You bet! Dandelion aids in controlling blood sugar and digestion. Chive flowers are delicious. Rose is rich in vitamin C, which can enhance the immune system. All three of these flowers can be used dried, strained, and enjoyed as a tea.

Borage, daisies, marigold, and violets are some of my favorites. You can grow edible flowers yourself—but stay clear of ones sprayed with pesticides. Or, do as I do, and order a garden-variety of dried edible flowers online: Try organic lavender flowers, dried: For tea, lemonade, and baking. Edible pansies for cake and cupcake toppers.

Crystallized Flowers

If you're looking for a simple recipe for you to put to use for serving the perfect flowers in perfect form—you've got it. Mix 1 cup flowers, 1 egg white, ½ cup sugar. Add egg white in small shallow bowl, beat lightly. In another bowl add sugar. Using a tiny new clean paint brush, paint flower of petals on both sides with egg white, until all coated. Over bowl with sugar, sprinkle both sides of flower or petal using a spoon, until all coated. Place on a wire rack over waxed paper, let dry. Garnish desserts or salads.

(Courtesy: Gemma Sanita Sciabica, *Cooking with California Olive Oil: Popular Recipes*)

HOMEMADE POTPOURRI RECIPES

Some folks believe potpourri is a trend from the seventies and sort of a thing of the past. Not so. Sure, it's not found in every household bathroom, drawers, or bedroom on a nightstand. But potpourri still has its place in the household.

There are a lot of store-bought potpourri concoctions available online. They are perfect in looks and most likely fragrant, too. But like uniform cookies, when you make them yourself the gift is that rustic appeal. Personally, I love to put dried and fresh herbs and spices in a pot on the stove and let it simmer. Each season I use a different recipe to provide scents to give the home a fresh scent.

Here, take a look at some potpourri concoctions you can do yourself in your kitchen and enjoy throughout the house, season by season.

Wintertime Spice Potpourri: In a pot, combine 1 grapefruit, sliced with peel, 1 lemon, sliced with peel, 2 cinnamon sticks, 2 teaspoons cloves, whole or powder, 2 teaspoons nutmeg, 2 teaspoons allspice. In a pan, combine all ingredients. Fill with water ¾ to the top. Simmer for 20 minutes. Turn off heat and enjoy the fragrance of winter spices. When cool put in container and cover. Store in refrigerator. Use for a few days. Simply pour into pot and simmer on the stovetop to provide aromatherapy in the kitchen.

Springtime Fresh Potpourri: In a sachet bag (available online) fill it up with spring dried herbs. Combine 2 teaspoons each dried lemon peels, parsley, and thyme. Add star anise for the presentation. Place in a mason jar. Close and open when you need a pick-me-up for feeling rejuvenated.

Summer Cool Potpourri: Use a large open seashell. In a pan combine cooling ¼ cup dried orange citrus peels, 4 tablespoon dried mint leaves, and 2 teaspoons dried parsley. Add ¼ cup small pebbles or shells and ¼ cup star anise. Leave out in the bathroom. Note: Place in a high region to keep children and pets away from the mixture.

Autumn Bliss Potpourri: In a ceramic dish, add 2 tablespoons each of cloves (whole), nutmeg, and pumpkin spice. Add ½ cup pine bark chips (available online), add a few mini pinecones. Leave on a dining room or living room table. Note: Place in a high region to keep children and pets away from the mixture.

Grounding
365 Herbal Potpourri

The draw of colors and symbols of herbs and spices goes back centuries. Here's proof: Herbal folk legends say putting bay leaves nearby you can help bring good luck and prosperity. I did it with crushed bay leaves and sprinkled the green herb on top of a note with my money wish. And yes, the bay leaf did work magic. Money matters changed. If you don't believe in the power of attraction, this recipe of mine will still titillate your nose 365 days a year.

6 ounces lavender flowers, dried
2 ounces marigold flowers, dried
2 ounces bay leaves, crushed or whole
2 ounces peppermint essential oil
10 drops lavender essential oil
10 drops lavender essential oil
10 drops rose essential oil

In a cedar wooden box with a top, combine all dry ingredients, flowers and leaves. Add essential oils. Mix well. Cover container. Store in a dark, cool, dry cupboard. After three days, remove the top and you have a fragrant spring potpourri. Dried flowers and essential oils are available online.

Safety Sound Bite: Put in a place where children and pets cannot reach the mixture.

It's time.Now you get to sweet stuff—like a chewy roll in a tootsie pop. I've collected a garden-variety of ways toenjoy herbs and spices year-round. The exciting tips I'm eager to share will help you to add spice to your life, year after year.

HEALING HIGHLIGHTS FROM NATURE'S GARDEN-FEST

✓ Herbs and spices have been used indoors and outdoors for centuries by people around the globe.
✓ Not only do they provide aromatic comfort and ambiance in the kitchen and all rooms of a household, gardens are a healing oasis.
✓ Yes, herbs and spices can make cuisine flavorful and fragrant but they also provide health benefits.
✓ Learning how to create home gifts, such as herbal wreaths for all seasons and spicy potpourri year-round, can morph a house into a home with aromatic feel-good emotions, such as calming and energizing benefits.

✓ Enjoying a sustainable outdoor garden during spring and summer will provide a beautiful atmosphere . . . and you'll have green pesticide-free fresh herbs to add to dishes and beverages . . .

✓ . . . And in the autumn and winter when there is less sunshine, you still can enjoy an indoor garden with hardy fresh herbs for dishes . . . Use a windowsill or plant light.

PART 6

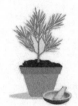

HERB-A-LICIOUS
RECIPES

Cooking It Up with Plants

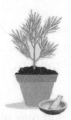

*Cookery means . . . English thoroughness, French art,
and Arabian hospitality. It means the knowledge of all
fruits and herbs and balms and spices; it means
carefulness, and watchfulness.*
—JOHN RUSKIN

I was ready to attend a book-signing adventure (first try) in Anchorage, Alaska—a state known for its link to nature's vibe. For my first night I planned to order a grilled corn salad with shallot, fresh herbs, capsicum, and soft boiled egg with a smoked paprika dressing. But, but, but . . . two days before leaving on a jet plane in early fall of 2016, rare hurricane-force winds upstaged my trip. I canceled. No herby salad for me. Disappointed, a few days later I made a salad with fresh herbs and spices to recover from my disappointment. I vowed, "One day I will reschedule the northern exposure escapade and order Alaskan fish and salad with fresh seasonings."

Four Seasons, Herbs and Spices

FALL

Autumn is a romantic time of the year. It's a time of change. The air is cooler, while colors of leaves on plants and trees turn earthy hues of gold and red. Cozy sweaters, jeans, and Uggs are part of warming up—like savoring the warm spices.

Herbal Foodstuff: It is a time when herbs and spices are used to give heat to a dish. Seasonings are warming and can be added to hearty hot soups, baked sandwiches, warm vegetable salads, and spicy apple crisps, herby breads, sweet and savory muffins, and pies.

Herbs and Spices: Cilantro, chives, clove, parsley, thyme, allspice, cardamom, nutmeg, apple spice, and pumpkin spice.

WINTER

On December 21, the days are shorter and nights are longer. The air is colder and comfort foods are welcoming. Usage of fresh herbs and spices depends on where you live. That's where dried seasonings come into play. Sure, fresh is best but spicing it up in the winter can be a godsend, too.

Herbal Foodstuff: Stews and casseroles are on the stovetop and in the oven. Pumpkin spice from autumn through the holiday season are in demand. Using the right herbs and spices (fresh or dried) for aroma, flavor, and healing powers throughout the season of hibernation are popular.

Herbs and Spices: Bay leaf, thyme, allspice, cardamom, herbes de Provence, nutmeg, and pumpkin spice.

SPRING

During springtime, which goes from late March through late June, the signs of renewal and life of herbs and spices start to sprout. That mean fresh leaves, buds, and flowers pop up with the promise of life and vibrant colors to some. Herbal gardens and wild herbs and edible flowers begin to blossom.

Herbal Foodstuff: Eating during spring is a time to detox, enjoy lighter foods and beverages, complemented by lighter herbs and spices—and edible flowers.

Herbs and Spices: Cilantro, chives, dill, garlic, marjoram, parsley, and turmeric.

SUMMER

The hottest season starts June 21. This is a popular time to nurture and savor a fresh home herb garden—and indoors by windowsills, too. It's time to enjoy flavorful plant-based dishes, like salads, cold soups, sandwiches, and smoothies—spiced up with herbs and spices. An abundance of fresh herbs are available at grocery stores and in our gardens.

Herbal Foodstuff: Hot and spicy seasonings are in demand with their ability to rev up metabolism and add flavor to the food herbivores love best.

Herbs and Spices: Cayenne, cilantro, dill, fennel, oregano, paprika, and tarragon.

Recipes (marked with an *) can be found in previous chapters, especially at the end of each one, or in the recipes section in the following chapter. You can mix and match to fit your personal taste and fit the season.

FALL

Breakfast:
French Toast*
Fresh autumn fruit
Spice-flavored coffee or tea

Lunch:
1 bowl Herbal Greek Bean Soup*
Cheese and Chive Scones with Herb Butter*

Snack:
Pot of herbal tea
1 square Pumpkin Spice Walnut Fudge*

Dinner:
Spicy Italian Meatballs*
Tossed Salad with Creamy Garlic Dressing*

Snack:
Herbal tea
1 slice Autumn Allspice Teacake*

WINTER

Breakfast:
1 bowl oatmeal with sliced apples, bananas, nuts, sprinkled with
    cinnamon-sugar, nutmeg, and allspice
1 cup herbal tea (winter spice)

Lunch:
Pasta with Garlic and Tomatoes*
1 cup vegetables

Snack:
1 cup spiced coffee

Dinner:
Beef Tenderloin with Chives and Parsley (Topped with Red Wine
    Demi Sauce) *
Kale salad with tomatoes, herbs, and spices
Pasta with thyme and pepper
Garlic toast

Snack:
Spicy Sweet Potato Pie*

SPRING

Breakfast:
Smoothie: Blend springtime fruits, organic milk, cinnamon, nutmeg, and allspice
1 cup herbal tea

Lunch:
Cilantro Lime Slaw*
Grilled cheese with tomatoes on whole grain bread sprinkled with ground pepper, basil

Snack:
Jumbo Anise Biscotti*
1 cup spiced coffee

Dinner:
Mediterranean Oven-Baked Garlic and Marjoram Pizza*
Tossed greens

Snack:
Grapes and slice of cheese with thyme sprigs
Herbal tea

SUMMER

Breakfast:
Scrambled Eggs with Chives and Goat Cheese*
Toast with cinnamon-sugar

Lunch:
1 piece of baked chicken or cold fried chicken
Dill-Lemon Potato Salad*

Snack:
1 glass lemonade: fresh lemons, water, honey or sugar to taste, parsley sprigs, and mint

Dinner:
Mussels Marina Sauce with Bay Leaf and Pasta*
Artichoke with mayonnaise and herbs of your choice
Cilantro Cheesy Pull-Apart Bread*

Snack:
Nutmeg Peach Crumble*
Iced tea with mint sprigs

ETHNIC CUISINE WITH SEASONINGS

Adventurous eating is exciting. The thrill comes with herbs and spices. If you have fish or vegetables it is bland without seasonings. Once you spice it up, the dish can titillate your taste buds and by savoring the food with a Mediterranean flair, Indian kick, or Spanish gusto. It changes the food to a different flavor and different aroma. Herbs and spices in your fare can whisk you around the globe in the comfort of your kitchen.

Here are some healthful choices to help you stay lean and heart-healthy. Each type of cuisine includes dishes that are laden with high fat—but why take that path? Take another route for your health's sake—and the herbs and spices will give you that exotic thrill. Caveat: Once in a while, give into your cravings for a decadent dish for a special occasion. If cooking at home, the herbs and spices will provide extra flavoring, whereas you may be able to use less fat, salt, and sugar.

French Best Choices: Endive and watercress salad, steamed fish, sautéed vegetables, chicken in wine sauce, French bread, fresh fruit.

Special Occasions: Croissants, cheeses, cheesecake, and quiche.

Herbs and Spices: Bay leaves, chives, garlic, marjoram, nutmeg, parsley, tarragon, and thyme.

Greek Best Choices: Tossed greens with tomatoes and feta cheese, a vegetable stew or soup, fresh fish with vegetables and rice.

Special Occasions: Lamb, Pork, fried foods.

Herbs and Spices: Dill, garlic, nutmeg, and oregano.

Indian: Bean dishes, tundori chicken and fish, pita bread, chicken kabobs, and yogurt cucumber salad.

Special Occasions: Dishes with peanut sauces, samosa (fried turnovers).

Herbs and Spices: Cardamom, cilantro, cloves, cumin, garlic, nutmeg, saffron, and turmeric.

Italian: Minestrone soup, pasta with marinara sauce, chicken cacciatore, pizza with fresh vegetable toppings, Italian bread, fresh fruit, skim milk with cappuccino.

Special Occasions: Meat ravioli, fried appetizers.

Herbs and Spices: Bay leaves, fennel seeds, garlic, marjoram, oregano, and parsley.

Spanish: Chicken fajitas, fish tacos, and tortillas with salsa.

Special Occasions: Enchiladas, refried beans.

Herbs and Spices: Cayenne, cumin, garlic, paprika, parsley, and saffron.

PAIRING PARTNERS, SEASONINGS

Now that you know which herbs and spices dish medicinal benefits, it's time to dish it up, the best ways. You can use herbs and spices solo, but pairing seasonings will give more bang for your buck and a double whammy of good-for-you healing compounds. Here's an at-a-glance pairing partners guide to help you get started when mixing and matching my herbs and spices for your palate's sake.

Herb and Spice	Perfect Pairings	Culinary Uses
Allspice	Cardamom, cloves	Baking
Anise	Cardamom, nutmeg	Baking
Bay leaf	Parsley, thyme	Cooking
Caraway	Dill, fennel, garlic, oregano	Baking/cooking

Herb and Spice	Perfect Pairings	Culinary Uses
Cardamom	Cloves, nutmeg	Baking/cooking
Cayenne	Cumin, cilantro, dill, garlic	Cooking
Chives	Dill, parsley, tarragon	Cooking
Cilantro	Cumin, fennel, garlic, oregano	Cooking
Cloves	Cardamom, nutmeg, star anise	Baking
Cumin	Cilantro, garlic, parsley	Cooking
Dill	Caraway, chives, parsley, tarragon	Cooking
Fennel	Cilantro, garlic, oregano, parsley	Cooking
Garlic	Cilantro, chives, parsley, oregano	Cooking
Marjoram	Parsley, thyme	Cooking
Nutmeg	Allspice, clove, cumin	Baking
Oregano	Cumin, fennel, garlic, parsley	Cooking
Paprika	Garlic, parsley	Cooking
Parsley	Bay leaf, chives, dill, garlic, thyme	Cooking
Saffron	Bay leaf, chives, cloves, fennel	Cooking/baking
Tarragon	Garlic, thyme	Cooking
Thyme	Bay leaf, dill, oregano, parsley	Cooking
Turmeric	Garlic, parsley	Cooking

SAVVY SEASONED TIPS FOR COOKING

Here is an herbs and spices at-a-glance chart just for you. It shares know-how of culinary herbs and spices.

Herb and Spice Chart

chef-menus.com/herb_and_spice_chart.html

Fresh Herbs - Flavor and Uses		Spices - Form, Flavor, and Uses	
Basil	Sweet, sunny flavor versatile. Green beans, peas potatoes, chicken dishes, tomato sauces, salads. Only add at end of cooking time or on prepared dish	**Allspice**	*Berries, ground.* Similar to cloves and cinnamon combo, more complex. Cakes, cookies, relishes, tomato sauce, stew, chicken, lamb
Bay Leaves	Pungent, mint like; dried leaves more widely available. Used in sauces, stews, gumbos; many varieties	**Celery**	*Seeds, ground.* Stronger than celery flavor. Salad dressings, potatoes, veggies, soups, beans, pork
Chives	Delicate onion flavor, never overpowering. Use at end of cooking or as final flavor garnish. Chop finely; snip with scissors. Great with eggs, salads, potatoes dishes, poultry, sauces	**Chile Peppers**	*Ground, dried whole, pepper flakes.* Made by grinding hot chilies. Countless types from many countries. Mild to blistering hot. Soups, stews, beans, sauces, poultry, greens; add to most foods for that extra kick
Cilantro	Fresh, aromatic, distinctive. Predominate in Mexican and Chinese cookery; salsas, chutneys, chicken, pork, salads, tacos	**Chile Powder**	*Ground mixture* commonly of chile peppers, paprika, cumin, black pepper. Spicy, hot or mild. Chili, beans, Mexican dishes. Buy high-quality

1/4

Dill	Pungent, tangy; dominate, use alone or with parsley. Seeds also have strong flavor. Salmon, peas, eggplant, cabbage, cucumber yogurt sauces, salads, pickling; predominate in Mediterranean cooking	**Cinnamon**	*Sticks/bark, ground.* Pungent, sweet, hot. Fruit desserts, cakes cookies. Also try on pork, lamb, meat pies, curries
Marjoram	Oregano like but sweeter. Fish stews, "stuffings", carrots, greens, beans, egg dishes	**Cloves**	*Whole or ground.* Aromatic, sweet. Fruits, desserts, meats, curry, soups, beans, pork
Mint	Strong; sweet. Varieties include peppermint and spearmint. Teas, desserts, lamb, fish, salads. Good in Thai and other Asian dishes	**Cumin**	*Seeds, ground.* Bold, distinctive; can overpower. Chili, tacos, stews, cabbage, beans. Toast ground or seeds
Oregano	Earthy. Lamb, chicken, pork, seafood, eggplant, tomato sauces; excellent with lemon. Retains good flavor when dried	**Curry**	*Ground.* Mixture of numerous spices including cloves and cumin. Buy high-quality. Base spice for curries; use also in tomato sauces, stews
Parsley	Clean bright flavor. Good with almost any savory food; all seafood, beef, chicken, potatoes, sauces, soups, salads. Fresh is better than dried	**Fennel**	*Seeds, ground.* Licorice-like, stronger then fresh fennel. Bread, fish, Italian dishes, sausage, tomato sauces. Toast ground or seeds to enhance flavor

Rosemary	Fresh, piney, pungent; easily overpowers. Chop finely and use lightly. A must with poultry, potatoes, white beans, lamb, breads, fruit salads	**Ginger**	*Fresh root, ground, candied.* Pungent, spicy. Grate, mince to use in chicken, squash, sesame noodles, applesauce, chutneys, marinade. Ground and fresh have much different flavors. Predominate in Asian cooking
Sage	Almost mint-like, slightly bitter; can overpower other herbs. Use whole stems in soups, stews, remove when done. Chop whole leaves in very thin strips. Pork, veal, sausages, poultry, stuffing, sauces. Dried herb has much different flavor	**Mustard**	*Seeds, ground.* Often hot, pungent. Several varieties available. Vegetables, stews, relishes, seafood, salad dressings. Seeds can be toasted to enhance flavor.
Savory	Reminiscent of thyme. Veal, pork, eggplant tomatoes, stuffing	**Nutmeg**	*Whole, ground.* Sweet, spicy, fragrant. Cakes, fruit, desserts, beans, sauces, cabbage, spinach
Tarragon	Licorice, lemon flavor; strong. Use alone or with parsley; veal, chicken, potatoes, mushrooms, tomato dishes, vinaigrettes	**Paprika**	*Ground.* Made from red peppers. Can be mild or hot and pungent. Not just for garnish. Buy high-quality with fresh peppery aroma. Seafood, vegetables, eggs; almost anything

| Thyme | Earthy, subtle, versatile; use whole sprigs in soups, stews. Pluck leaves and add at all stages of cooking. Excellent in most dishes especially seafood, poultry, pork, veal, tomato, vegetables, breads. Retains good flavor when dried | Pepper | *Whole berries, ground.* Most common of all spices. Hot peppers, sweet peppers and peppercorns are from same plant. Peppercorns are black, white and green—depends on level of maturity. Pink peppercorns are a distant relative. Use on everything including sweets and fruits. Buy a pepper mill and whole peppercorns. You'll be glad you did! |

NOTES ON SHELF LIFE OF SEASONINGS

Fresh, dried, and homegrown herbs can be used and stored many ways. No, you cannot keep seasonings forever because they do lose their aroma, flavor, color, texture, and healing powers. So, here is a quick look at how to keep your favorite seasonings good to go every season!

Fresh Herbs: These are fabulous but the shelf life of herbs past their sell-by date is short. If you are lucky enough to have an herb garden, you'll have your pick during its season. As a Californian, we do have an abundance of fresh organic packaged herbs available at the grocery store. These herbs are freshest on the best-used-before date. Tick tock. I was surprised to discover many of my social media friends told me they not only take care of dried herbs but they preserve fresh herbs. How? How do they do it? Simply put, they freeze chopped herbs by putting them in plastic bags. Also, some folks combine the herbs with H_2O and freeze them in an ice cube tray.

As a Californian, we are blessed to have an abundance of fresh herbs, whether it be in our own gardens, grocery stores, or the farmers' market. However, I have wasted a lot of cilantro, parsley, and thyme, thinking, "I'll use it tomorrow"—sooner than later, it expired.

Dried Herbs: Enter dried herbs. I used to be a snob and only used fresh herbs. Nowadays, my collection of dried herbs is plentiful. It provides convenience and variety. Dried herbs are wonderful because they're always there when you need them. So, how long do dried herbs last? If you properly store them in a dark, cool pantry, the shelf life of herbs is about six months. Some brands, like McCormick, put a best-before date on their dried herbs. You can test to see if your dried herbs are still good by rubbing a bit of the herb in your hands. If there is good aroma, it's likely good. If you don't smell much you won't get much flavor or health benefits from using the dried herbs. Herbalists will tell you whole herbs (and spices like cloves and ginger) have the longest shelf life because they have not been exposed to air.

Spices: Dried spices like dried herbs must be stored in containers (glass or tin), away from heat or light or moisture. Like dried herbs there is often a best-used-before date. If you have a collection you put together, like I did, on the labels of each spice add the expiration date so you toss and replenish. Also, once opened it doesn't matter as long as you seal the container after usage.

When to Use Fresh and Dried Herbs and Spices: The rule of thumb is, you bake with dried herbs and spices. Use fresh sprigs or leaves to garnish. When cooking you can use some dried herbs, such as bay leaf, throughout the heating process like in a soup or sauce. Spices such as cardamom and nutmeg do fine throughout baking, such as in a cake or custard. Garnishing with fresh herbs is a nice touch.

Heart-Healthy

Oven-Baked Herbed Alaskan Salmon

Two months before departing on my second attempted trip to Anchorage, I had Alaskan salmon garnished with fresh herbs on the brain. Baked salmon (which I do eat on occasion) is rich in omega-3 fatty acids, which are heart-healthy and have anti-inflammatory benefits. My plans included feasting on that special dinner of Great Alaskan salmon with fresh garlic and thyme. Then, a shallow, widely felt 7.0 major earthquake rocked Anchorage. I canceled my book signing and booked flight due to thousands of aftershocks. So, I created this herby fish recipe for the trip that tanked.

1 lemon, sliced
8 ounces salmon, fillet
¼ cup European-style butter
2 tablespoons fresh garlic, minced
Ground lemon black pepper to taste (Mount Rose
    Herbs)
Fresh parsley and thyme sprigs

Preheat the oven to 350 degrees F. Cut lemon, place slices on foil. Season salmon with butter–garlic spice mixture. Slice fish in two pieces. Sprinkle with lemon pepper. Put fish on foil on a baking sheet or dish. Bake until fish is cooked and flaky, about 15 minutes. Serve with parsley and thyme sprigs, and sliced lemon. Serve on top a bed of wild rice.

Serves 3.

HEALING HIGHLIGHTS FROM NATURE'S GARDEN-FEST

✓ Chicken or fish, anyone? Spice it up with herbs and spices. You can have different cuisines, like Italian, Greek, Spanish dishes—it's all because of the seasonings you use.

✓ Using seasonings for the four seasons is a way to feel Earth changes throughout the year. Go ahead, use the right seasoning for the right season and get a JOLT OF ADVENTURE.

✓ Storing dried and fresh herbs and spices is key to preserving the flavor and health perks of seasonings.

✓ Season your foods for taste, texture, and presentation—but don't overpower a dish with one seasoning. Balance your herbs and spices for premium flavor and health.

Herbs and Spices Menu

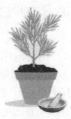

Oh better no doubt is a dinner of herbs,
When season'd with love which no rancor disturbs
And sweeten'd by all that is sweet in life
Than turbot, bisque, or tolans, eaten in strife!
—EDWARD BULWER-LYTTON (1831–1891), *Lucile*

I booked another flight for early winter to Anchorage, Alaska, because like tasting different herbs and spices—it promised an exciting experience. Before my journey I scrutinized a popular hotel food menu. It was my dream to feast on seasoned fresh salads, pastas, and fresh citrus fruit for breakfast in my suite overlooking the city skyline and snow-capped mountains.

Like always, my carry-on was filled with herbal teas, such as chamomile and hibiscus since I didn't get a flu shot. Alas, I did fulfill my dream of flying to Alaska! However, on a 737-800 jet, rough air due to the hurricane-force winds in Anchorage was nerve-racking. While we landed in Anchorage (not diverted to Fairbanks), I was greeted with no snow, fog with zero visibility, and cloud cover so no aurora borealis to view in the sky. The worst part? Garden-fresh organic herbs (like chefs at spas and on television love to use in cooking) are not readily available in December. But dried herbs and spices did come to the rescue. In this section, I do dish up recipes complete with fresh food, both fresh and dried herbs and spices, to enjoy in the comfort of your home, wherever you are and whatever the season.

THE RECIPES

The categories will include breakfasts, appetizers and sides, soups and salads, entrées, and desserts. Flavorful, adventurous, and timeless food trends (i.e., smoothies, slow cookers, power bowls, plant-based dishes) will be part of the herbal menu. Cooks at health spas, restaurants, cafés, and food trucks to celeb chefs on television, adore using herbs and spices. The Golden Door, for instance, has offered Fennel and Monkfish, Gold Carrot and Orange Soup with Cumin, Garlic-Herb Baguette, and Savory Five-Spice Tuiles. I will include delicious recipes, much like these, that you can enjoy.

BREAKFAST

They say breakfast is the most essential meal of the day. After fasting and not eating after 7:00 P.M. like Europeans do, I'm not famished first thing when I wake up. A quality cup of coffee with a splash of organic milk, fortified O.J., and whole grain cereal are familiar breakfast foods for me. But that doesn't mean I don't appreciate a cinnamon roll with spices or eggs with fresh herbs. A Cheese and Chive Scone, slice of Pumpkin Spicy Chocolate Chip Bread, or Spiced Biscotti served with chilled fresh squeezed fruit juice and a cup of tea is a continental breakfast from heaven.

Cheese and Chive Scones with Herb Butter
Cinnamon Rolls with Allspice Glaze
Olive Oil Vegetable Frittata with
Roasted Asparagus & Tomatoes
Scrambled Eggs with Spinach, Chives, & Goat Cheese
Zesty Pumpkin Chocolate Chip Bread

Cheese and Chive Scones
with Herb Butter

On a trip to Ontario, Canada, I was excited to be in a foreign country. I had visited the province decades prior. This time around, my experience was different. Before swimming in the hotel pool, I found myself at a coffee shop. Peering through the glass counter at pastries, the cheese and chive scones caught my eye. The counter girl was friendly. "I'll take a scone," I said, and pointed to the rectangle with green herbs. "Are you from the states?" she asked, and I laughed asking, "How did you know that?" We talked about homesickness and scones—a universal comfort food. There's something about warm scones and hot tea that is soothing. The fresh, warm scone was tasty with notes of mild onion-like-tasting chives. I fantasized about baking a batch once in my kitchen, with a backdrop of pine trees and my companion animals. This recipe is Canada-inspired with flavors from fresh herbs in Northern California.

2¾ cups self-rising flour
6 tablespoons European-style butter, cold, cubed
½ cup buttermilk
½ cup cheddar cheese, shredded
2 tablespoons chives, dried
¼ cup walnuts, chopped (optional)
1 egg, whisked

Preheat the oven to 350 degrees F. In a bowl, combine flour and butter. Add buttermilk, mix well. Fold in cheese and chives. Add walnuts if desired. On a cutting board, dust with flour. Place dough on it and form into a circle. Knead several times. Cut in half, repeat until you have 6 to 8 triangles. Place on parchment-lined cookie sheet. Brush with egg wash. Bake for about 15 to 20 minutes or until scones are lightly golden brown.

Serves 6.

HERB BUTTER

½ cup European-style butter
1 teaspoon parsley, fresh
1 teaspoon chives, fresh
1 teaspoon thyme, fresh

In a small bowl, mix soft butter with parsley, chives, and thyme. Herbs can be bought in the produce aisle at the store or homegrown. Chill in refrigerator until serving with Cheese and Chive Scones and herbal tea.

Cinnamon Rolls with Allspice Glaze

I have adapted this recipe from a combination of my collection. Truth be told, I have used store-bought dough and baked semi-rolls but it's almost as easy to make rolls from scratch. This version is sweet and spicy. Serve warm—with tea. It's a gift from nature's herbal garden.

DOUGH

2¼ cups self-rising flour and a bit extra to dust the cutting board
¼ cup granulated white sugar
¼ cup European-style butter, and a bit to grease the baking dish

FILLING

½ cup brown sugar
¼ cup granulated white sugar
¼ cup European-style butter, melted
1½ tablespoons ground cinnamon

¼ teaspoon cardamom
½ cup cranberries, dried and pecans, mixed

TOPPING

¼ cup ground cinnamon-sugar (Mountain Rose Herbs)

GLAZE

1 cup confectioners sugar
4 to 6 tablespoons half-and-half or whole milk
1 teaspoon vanilla extract
½ teaspoon ground allspice (McCormick)

Preheat the oven to 350 degrees F. In a bowl combine flour and sugar. Add soft butter and mix well. Turn out on a floured cutting board. Shape into a circle. Knead until there are no rough edges and dough is smooth. Use rolling pin to shape dough into a long rectangle. Set aside. In a bowl mix sugar, butter, cinnamon, cardamom, cranberries, and nuts. Spread mixture on the rectangle. Roll up the rectangle away from you until it's sealed. Use a sharp knife and cut into slices. Place each pinwheel on an 8-inch by 8-inch buttered square baking dish. Sprinkle tops with cinnamon-sugar. Bake for about 30 minutes or until light golden brown.

Cool, then drizzle with glaze or melt ½ cup honey with ¼ cup butter and use. Or not. These rolls are flavorful plain. Store for several days in the refrigerator or freeze and warm up in the microwave. Tip: Using self-rising flour is the twenty-first-century miracle. You can forget yeast, time, and baking powder while your herbal delights still rise! These cinnamon rolls are naturally sweet and savory. They are flaky, buttery, and best served warm to taste the spice notes. The nutty crunch and chewy cranberries are a nice touch. Pair with home-squeezed grapefruit or orange juice. Savor a spicy cinnamon roll year-round.

Makes 12 to 15.

Olive Oil Vegetable Frittata with Roasted Asparagus & Tomatoes

❖ ❖ ❖

Welcome to a frittata that is filled with herbs, including garlic, red pepper, parsley, and basil. It is created with heart-healthy olive oil and filled with vegetables. Studies have shown, notes the North American Olive Oil Association, that your body absorbs nutrients from greens and vegetables such as tomatoes better when they are consumed with a monounsaturated fat like olive oil! This recipe is one that is worth the time and results. It's a beautiful egg vegetable dish to serve for breakfast or brunch year-round.

6 large eggs, beat with 1 tablespoon water
2 tablespoons + garnish Parmesan Reggiano, grated
1 teaspoon garlic, minced
2 teaspoons shallot, small diced
1 roasted red pepper, peeled, deseeded, and diced
1 cup russet potatoes, peeled, small diced, boiled until
   tender, drained and chilled
1 tablespoon parsley, chopped
1 tablespoon basil, chopped
3 tablespoons extra virgin olive oil
1 cup cremini mushroom, sliced
¼ cup Fontina cheese
6 portions Roasted Asparagus* (recipe), four large
   stalks per portion
6 portions Roasted Tomatoes* (recipe), 2¼ wedges per
   portion

Beat eggs with water and then beat Parmesan into the egg mixture and reserve. Combine garlic, shallot, roasted pepper, potato, parsley, and basil and set aside. Heat extra virgin olive oil in a 12-inch nonstick sauté pan over high heat. Add mushrooms and sauté until they start to brown. Reduce heat to medium and add the reserved vegetable mixture. Sauté for about 1½ minutes. Season with salt and pepper to taste. Add a little additional olive oil if needed then add the reserved egg mixture to the hot sauté pan.

Cook 2 to 3 minutes until egg cooks and sets on the bottom. Transfer the sauté pan to the broiler and broil until light and fluffy and almost totally set, about 2 to 3 minutes. Sprinkle Fontina cheese on top of the frittata and place back under the broiler just until melted, about 2 to 3 minutes. Remove to a cutting board and cut into 6 triangle servings. Place one serving into the center of the plate. Garnish each frittata portion with four stalks of hot roasted asparagus and two wedges of roasted tomato. Sprinkle each portion with Parmesan.

Serves 6.

(Courtesy: North American Olive Oil Association)

Scrambled Eggs With Spinach, Chives, & Goat Cheese

This egg recipe is quick and healthy. It's a gift from a chef's collected works. Sure, I include one of my own egg recipes, but this one is rich in superfoods—spinach—and is highlighted with goat cheese and chives. What's not to love? It's fresh for springtime—and can work year-round for breakfast, dinner, or a late-night snack.

6 cups fresh spinach
16 eggs (brown)
1 teaspoon salt
⅛ teaspoon black pepper
2 tablespoons olive oil
4 ounces goat cheese
2 tablespoon chives, chopped

Blanch spinach in salted boiling water. Drain in colander and cool under cold running water. Squeeze out excess liquid and chop. Beat the eggs well and season with salt and pepper. In a sauté pan over medium heat add the olive oil and eggs. Cook until eggs begin to set. Add spinach, cheese, and chives and continue cooking until eggs are set—but still soft. Serve hot.

Serves 8.

(Courtesy: Chef Ann Foundation)

Zesty Pumpkin Chocolate Chip Bread

A popular Vermont-based chocolate company's staff will tell you October is the perfect time of year for baking! Here are my words about their spicy bread recipe: This Pumpkin Chocolate Chip Bread recipe is a favorite of mine during autumn. It's a delicious and versatile bread for breakfast with a cup of joe to an afternoon treat with tea. It's a fall must-have for you and yours.

Autumn is my favorite season of the year, whether I'm in the sierras or traveling to Northeast Canada where the foliage colors are breathtaking. This spicy bread includes cayenne, cinnamon, and nutmeg—paired with a cup of hot herbal tea it's sure to please.

1 cup pumpkin puree
2 large eggs
½ cup vegetable oil
1⅓ cups granulated sugar
⅓ cup water
1 teaspoon vanilla extract
1¼ cups all-purpose flour
1 teaspoon baking soda
¼ teaspoon baking powder

½ *teaspoon nutmeg*
¾ *teaspoon salt*
¾ *cups chocolate (we recommend our Dark Spicy*
   Aztec Chocolate Bar, includes cayenne pepper and
   cinnamon) or 72 percent extra-dark chocolate bar
Pumpkin seeds or nuts (optional)

Preheat the oven to 350 degrees F. Lightly grease and flour a 9-inch by 5-inch loaf pan. In a large bowl, beat together the pumpkin puree, eggs, oil, sugar, water, and vanilla. Add the flour, baking soda, baking powder, nutmeg, and salt, stirring just to combine. Fold in chopped chocolate and pour into the prepared loaf pan. Bake for 50 to 60 minutes, or until a cake tester comes out clean. Cool on a rack for about 30 minutes, then tip out of the pan and cool completely on the rack. Wrap tightly and store in a cool, dry place. Makes 1 loaf. For best results, store overnight before serving to allow the flavors and texture to develop.

(Author's recommendation. Add 1 teaspoon pumpkin spice or allspice to the batter.)

Serves 8 to 10.

(Courtesy: Lake Champlain Chocolates)

APPETIZERS AND SIDES

Introduction bites and side dishes can often upstage the entrée or dessert, especially if special attention is given to herbs and spices. Seasoning can give food aroma, flavor, and better presentation. It can make food have its own imprint. Deviled Crab Cakes with a Creole Seasoning can make it a Cajun delight. Zucchini Sticks with Herbal Dip scream West Coast and can be layered with Mediterranean notes.

During a trip to Victoria, British Columbia, I enjoyed the concierge room, which served appetizers in the late afternoon. The array of crackers, olives, cheese, and fresh fruit inspired me to make a delightful cheese plate. Once put together I was too full to order in or go out to eat. But herbs and spices were missing. Back home, I often do a redo and add fresh herbs to the food. So, an appetizer or side can be a winner, wherever you are, especially if seasoned with special TLC from home.

Couscous with Apricots and Toasted Cumin
Deviled Crab Cakes
Garlic EVVO Smashed Potatoes and Parsnips
Herbed Cornbread and Thyme Stuffing
Shrimp and Wild Rice Cakes with Roasted Pepper-Dill Aioli
Spicy Roasted Vegetables
Zucchini Sticks with Herbal Dip

Couscous with Apricots and Toasted Cumin

❖ ❖ ❖

After viewing the past award-winning film *Leaving Las Vegas*, I was amused by Nicholas Cage's character Ben who put too much salt on his spaghetti. This is a recipe worth dishing up—and it does include a bit of salt. The herbs and spices give it plenty of flavor, too. (Food Network judges often note chefs need to include salt because it brings out the best zest in foods.)

2 cups water
1 package plain couscous (I used 10 ounces, uncooked)
½ cup coarsely chopped dried apricots
2 plum tomatoes, coarsely chopped
½ cup finely chopped fresh parsley
¼ cup thinly sliced green onions
2 teaspoons McCormick Gourmet Organic Cumin, ground
¼ teaspoon McCormick Gourmet Organic Coriander, ground
¼ cup lemon juice
¼ cup olive oil
1 tablespoon honey
1 teaspoon McCormick Gourmet Sicilian Sea Salt
1 teaspoon McCormick Gourmet Organic Black Pepper, coarse ground
1 cup toasted slivered almonds

Bring water to boil in medium saucepan on high heat. Stir in couscous and apricots. Remove from heat; cover. Let stand 5 minutes or until liquid has been absorbed. Fluff with a fork. Spoon into large bowl. Cool about 10 minutes, tossing occasionally with a fork. Add tomatoes, parsley, and green onions; toss to mix well.

Meanwhile, cook and stir cumin and coriander in small dry skillet on medium heat 2 to 3 minutes or until fragrant and darker in color. Pour into small bowl. Stir in lemon juice, oil, honey, sea salt, and pepper with wire whisk until well blended. Add dressing and almonds to couscous mixture; toss to coat well. Serve at room temperature or refrigerate until ready to serve.

Serves 8.

(Courtesy: McMcormick)

Deviled Crab Cakes

I've had crabmeat served in fancy salads, and as a child who spent part of every summer at Santa Cruz beach, I ate a lot of fish. Fish and chips served on the boardwalk and wharf was my favorite. This herb-a-licious baked crab cakes recipe is similar to my mother's "adult" version of tuna fish croquettes.

3 tablespoon unsalted butter
¼ cup onion, minced
¼ cup bell pepper, minced
3 tablespoons celery, minced
1 large egg
1 tablespoon sour cream
1 teaspoon salt
1 tablespoon King Creole seasoning (The Spice House)
¼ teaspoon Worcestershire powder
½ teaspoon dry mustard
½ pound jumbo lump or backfin crabmeat
2 tablespoons green onion, minced
16 saltines, crushed
Vegetable oil, enough for sautéing patties

Melt the butter in a sauté pan, sauté the onion, bell pepper, and celery until tender. Set aside. In a large bowl, whisk together the egg, sour cream, and spices. Stir in the crabmeat, sautéed vegetables, green onion, and half of the saltine crumbs. Mix thoroughly. Form into 2-inch patties and coat with the remaining saltine crumbs. Sauté in vegetable oil until golden brown [about 15 minutes or until crisp].

Serves 4.

(Courtesy: The Spice House)

Garlic EVVO Smashed Potatoes and Parsnips

Mashed potatoes are a staple side dish, especially during Thanksgiving and Christmas. Instead of making the same old taters with gravy, why not change it up with the gift of garlic? You'll want to add this herby recipe to your favorite picks and for the picky eaters who don't love parsnips.

Garlic Olive Oil

1 head of garlic (washed and dried)
½ cup extra virgin olive oil
Preheat the oven to 250 to 300 degrees F. Split the garlic head in half to expose cloves. In small loaf pan, cover garlic heads with extra virgin olive oil. Place foil over pan and put in oven until garlic is fully cooked and soft. Remove garlic heads and pop out cloves. Strain extra virgin olive oil to remove skins. Puree cooked cloves with strained oil.

Garlic Extra Virgin Olive Oil Mashed Potatoes and Parsnips

3 medium to large russet potatoes, peeled and diced
3 large parsnips, peeled and diced

3 tablespoons parsley, thinly shredded (chiffonade)
Garlic olive oil to taste
Salt and pepper to taste

Combine potatoes and parsnips in water. Boil until tender. Drain well. In a large roasting pan smash drained potatoes and parsnips with a fork. Season hot potatoes and parsnips with parsley, garlic oil, salt, and pepper. Serve immediately.

Serves 6.

(Courtesy: North American Olive Oil Association)

Herbed Cornbread and Thyme Stuffing

I picked up this recipe for stuffing in the twenty-first century in my mountain cabin. It's a bit spicier than some versions I've made—but it's delightful. I do not eat hens, turkey, or chicken—but I relish the cornbread, vegetables, and herbs. No fowl needed.

¼ cup European-style butter
1 onion, yellow, diced
2 teaspoons garlic, minced
¾ cup mushrooms, rinsed, chopped
1 cup store-bought cornbread, cubes or crumbled
½ teaspoon marjoram, dried
½ teaspoon thyme, dried
1 teaspoon herbes de Provence (Mountain Rose Herbs)
1 tablespoon European-style butter (for greasing baking dish)
Fresh thyme sprigs

In a nonstick frying pan, melt butter on medium heat. Add onion, garlic, and mushrooms. Sauté ingredients for a few several minutes. Fold in cornbread, marjoram, thyme, and herbes de Provence. Put in a butter-greased baking dish or individual ramekins. Follow cornbread package directions for baking time and oven temperature. Garnish with thyme.

Serves 4 to 6.

Shrimp and Wild Rice Cakes with Roasted Pepper-Dill Aioli

❖ ❖ ❖

ROASTED PEPPER-DILL AIOLI

1 cup light mayonnaise
1 jar (7 ounces) roasted red peppers, finely chopped
½ teaspoon McCormick Gourmet Organic Dill Weed
½ teaspoon McCormick Gourmet Organic Mustard, Ground
¼ teaspoon McCormick Gourmet Organic Garlic Powder
¼ teaspoon McCormick Gourmet Organic Black Pepper, Coarse Ground

SHRIMP AND WILD RICE CAKES

½ cup flour
1 teaspoon baking powder
1 teaspoon Old Bay Seasoning
1 cup chopped cooked shrimp
¼ cup chopped green onions
½ cup cooked (unsalted) wild rice
¾ teaspoon McCormick Gourmet Organic Dill Seed
¾ teaspoon McCormick Gourmet Organic Thyme

¼ *cup (½ stick) butter, melted*
¼ *cup milk*
2 eggs, beaten

For the Aioli, mix all ingredients in medium bowl; cover. Refrigerate until ready to serve.

For the Shrimp Cakes, mix flour, baking powder, and Old Bay in large bowl. Stir in shrimp, green onions, cooked rice, dill seed, and thyme. Add butter, milk, and eggs; gently stir until well blended. Spray large nonstick skillet with no-stick cooking spray. Heat on medium heat. Drop heaping teaspoonfuls of shrimp mixture into skillet. Flatten slightly so cakes are about 2 inches in diameter. Cook cakes in small batches, 5 minutes per side, or until lightly browned. Serve shrimp cakes with half of the Aioli. (Remaining Aioli may be used as a sandwich spread or as a dip for vegetables.)

Serves 12.

(Courtesy: McCormick)

Spicy Roasted Vegetables

❖ ❖ ❖

NOTE that the base for the spice blend is from Pasolivo, a popular olive oil ranch in California. Cooking vegetables isn't rocket science. But this recipe includes a superb mix of vegetables complemented with the right mix of spices. The blend includes almonds, macadamia nuts, pistachios, sesame seeds, coriander, cumin, and sea salt.

3 tablespoons Pasolivo Dukkah Blend
1 tablespoon Central Coast curry
1 tablespoon cumin
1 cup classic extra virgin olive oil
4 large onions, thinly sliced

1 large butternut squash, ¼ inch julienne
1 large yam or sweet potato, ¼ inch julienne
3 large parsnips, ¼ inch julienne
6 carrots, ¼ inch julienne
1 head cauliflower broken into small pieces

In a small bowl, mix the Pasolivo Dukkah Blend, Central Coast curry, and cumin. Put all of the ingredients in a large bowl and mix well. Pour onto two 18-inch by 13-inch sheet pans and spread evenly to cover the pans. Roast for 12 minutes or until tender and some edges are crisping and caramelizing.

[*One-half cup is a standard serving. If you use 1 cup paired with ¾ cup rice or pasta it can be a main dish.]

(Courtesy: Pasolivo)

Zucchini Sticks with Herbal Dip

One pre-summer I was craving an easy to make and healthful appetizer. In the fridge, my eyes were drawn to the fresh zucchini. "Ah, zucchini fries are perfect!" I thought. This recipe is inspired by my youthful days in San Jose. There was a popular artichoke shop, and fried artichokes were one of my favorite appetizers. But zucchini fries minus frying (you can use an egg with herb panko for a crispy crunch) with plenty of European herbs and spices makes it a vegetable feast for vegetarians.

2 large zucchinis
2 eggs
½ cup Parmesan cheese shavings
2 cups Italian seasoned panko breadcrumbs
1 teaspoon oregano
½ teaspoon garlic salt

¼ cup tablespoons European-style butter, melted
Ground pepper to taste
3 tablespoons parsley, fresh

Herbal Dip

½ cup plain Greek yogurt
½ cup sour cream
1 teaspoon garlic, fresh, minced
2 tablespoons fresh lemon juice
1 teaspoon dill, ground
Ground black pepper to taste

Preheat the oven to 350 degrees F. Wash zucchini, cut stems, slice in halves, repeat. Place pieces on a baking dish. Set aside. In a bowl, combine eggs and Parm cheese. Set aside. In a flat dish mix breadcrumbs and spices. Dip zucchini wedges into egg mixture, then roll into breadcrumb mix. Place wedges onto a baking pan. Drizzle zucchini with melted butter. Sprinkle with pepper. Bake at 400 degrees F. for about 20 minutes or until golden and crispy. Meanwhile, in a bowl, combine yogurt and sour cream. Mix well. Add garlic, lemon juice, dill, and pepper. Chill. Serve dip with hot zucchini sticks garnished with fresh parsley. You can also serve ½ cup ketchup mixed with 1 Roma tomato, chopped, and 2 tablespoons fresh cilantro.

Serves 4.

SALADS, SOUPS, AND SANDWICHES

A garden salad tossed with a garlic dressing is a light meal to me. A hearty Herbal Greek Bean Soup paired with fresh artisan bread can suffice for lunch or dinner. Eggs with Herbs on Toasted Bread can be an artful presentation for kids or adults. The bottom line: Eating salads and soups can be served before a dinner entrée or they can be savored as a meal itself. This line-up is full of herbs and spices and will satisfy you and yours year-round.

Cilantro Lime Slaw
Edible Wildflowers and Arugula Salad
Egg and Artichoke Salad with Tarragon
Herbal Greek Bean Soup
Eggs with Herbs on Whole Grain Toasted Bread
Tossed Salad with Creamy Garlic Dressing
Vegetable Shell Pasta Salad with Olives, Fennel, & Onions

Cilantro Lime Slaw

❖ ❖ ❖

Cilantro can be an acquired taste as it was for me. But, but, but if you mix it up with plenty of spices, vinegar, and flavored olive oil and serve it chilled—it may wow your palate. Try this simple but elegant slaw and wakey wakey your taste buds!

⅓ cup apple cider vinegar
⅓ cup Pasolivo Lime Olive Oil
3 tablespoons sugar
½ teaspoon salt
½ teaspoon black pepper
1 bunch cilantro
1 medium serrano pepper
1 head green cabbage
¼ cup of mayonnaise or to taste

Whisk vinegar, olive oil, sugar, salt, and pepper in a bowl. Add cilantro and serrano pepper. Cut cabbage into quarters then into strings. Add mayo to vinegar mixture until blended, then toss in cabbage to coat. Refrigerate for at least 45 minutes before serving. Toss a few times again before serving to meld the flavors.

Serves 8–10.

(Courtesy: Pasolivo)

Edible Wildflowers and Arugula Salad

My trip to Anchorage, Alaska, didn't include flowers and fresh herb salads. But if I lived there, I could have ordered online dried edible wildflowers. Here, an edible flower salad inspired by my cooking mentor Gemma Sciabica, who was dishing up flower dishes like this one back in the twentieth century the way people do now in the twenty-first century.

1½ cups curly endive, chopped
1 store-bought feta and herb cheese, crumbled
1 red pepper, roasted, chopped
2 cups arugula, chopped
¼ cup cilantro
4 sprigs thyme, chopped
¾ cup cherry tomatoes, chopped
1 cup edible flowers for garnish (I prefer pansies, found online)
½ cup seeds (pumpkin or sunflower)

In a bowl, combine all ingredients except the flowers. Set aside. In another bowl, whisk ½ cup olive oil and 2 teaspoons herbal vinegar (a ratio of 3 to 1 for oil and vinegar). Add minced garlic and lemon juice to taste. Garnish with flowers and sprinkle seeds on top. Drizzle with dressing.

Serves 2 as a main dish, 4 as a side dish.

Egg and Artichoke Salad with Tarragon
❖ ❖ ❖

You can spice up an egg salad with a French flair, and food author and judge Judy Ridgeway shows you how to do it. "Tarragon is just so good with eggs."

This combination of eggs, artichokes, and fresh tarragon comes from a simple restaurant in the French region of Brittany. The artichokes are essentially a Mediterranean vegetable, but 75 percent of the French production comes from this coastal area of northern France where they grow to a great size. You can cook and trim your own artichokes, but it is a good deal easier to buy canned artichokes bases.

8 large artichoke bases, canned or cooked and
*   prepared at home*
3 large eggs
¼ cup mayonnaise
2 tablespoons thick full fat yogurt
2 level tablespoons freshly chopped tarragon
2 teaspoons capers, roughly chopped
Freshly ground black pepper to taste
½ cucumber sliced

CARROT AND APPLE SALAD

1 large carrot, peeled and grated
1 tablespoon extra virgin olive oil
1 tablespoon fresh lemon juice
1 small apple, peeled, cored and cut into tiny cubes

Drain the canned artichoke hearts and soak in cold water for a while to remove any added salt. Hard boil the eggs and leave to stand in cold water until required. Skin the eggs and roughly chop. Mix the mayonnaise with the yogurt, tarragon, capers, and black pepper. Stir the eggs into the mayonnaise mixture and chill until serving. To make the carrot and apple salad, mix the grated carrot with olive oil and lemon juice and fold in the tiny cubes of apple. Place two artichoke bases on each plate and top with the egg and tarragon mixture. Arrange the carrot and apple salad at the side of the plate and garnish with sliced cucumber.

Serves 4.

(Courtesy: Judy Ridgway, Author and Judge)

Herbal Greek Bean Soup

On a cold winter day, a hearty soup chock-full of herbs like garlic and onion with spices such as paprika, pepper, and salt is perfect. This recipe for Fasolada is a traditional Greek soup made with white beans. You can make it in a slow cooker, but I prefer the old-fashioned method of stovetop.

1 pound dry white beans (Cannellini or Navy Beans)
1 large onion, diced
3 to 4 carrots, diced
3 stalks of celery, diced
2 cloves of garlic
2 tablespoons of olive oil
1 teaspoon paprika (hot or sweet)
1 (14.5 ounces) can diced tomatoes
½ cup extra virgin olive oil
Salt and pepper to taste

STOVETOP

If cooking on a stovetop, you must first soak the beans. Rinse the beans and pour into a large bowl. Cover with 2 inches of water, 1 tablespoon of salt, and let soak on the counter for 4 hours to 12 hours. In a large pot, starting with a cold pan, sauté the onion, carrots, celery, and garlic in 2 tablespoons of olive oil. When the vegetables are aromatic, add paprika. After 2 minutes, add the diced tomato and sauté for 1 minute. Add the soaked beans and cover with enough water to cover the beans by 1 inch. Season generously with salt. Simmer until the beans are tender (30 to 40 minutes). Add ½ cup of extra virgin olive oil and cook for a few more minutes. The olive oil will make the soup thick and creamy.

Slow Cooker

Rinse the beans. Add onion, celery, carrot, and garlic to the pot. If you can, sauté them first, but you don't have to. Add the paprika and the diced tomatoes. Add beans and enough water to cover by 1 inch. Add ½ cup of olive oil. Season generously with salt. Cook on high for 6 hours. Using a spoon, smash some of the beans to thicken the soup.

Instant Pot

Rinse the beans. Press the sauté button. Add 2 tablespoons of olive oil and sauté the onion, celery, carrots, and garlic. After 2 minutes, add the paprika. After 1 minute, add the diced tomato and sauté for 1 minute. Add the beans and enough water to cover by 1 inch. Press the cancel button to turn off the sauté mode. Press the manual button and adjust to 40 minutes. Make sure the pot is sealed. When done cooking, natural pressure release for 10 minutes or until the pressure pin drops. Open the pot and add ½ cup of olive oil. Stir. Put the machine back into sauté mode and let the soup simmer for 5 minutes.

To serve: Taste the soup and season with salt and pepper. Serve in bowl with crusty peasant bread, olives, and feta cheese! Enjoy and stay warm! This soup, like many soups and stews, tastes even better the next day.

Serves 6 to 8.

(Courtesy: North American Olive Oil Association)

Eggs with Herbs on Whole Grain Toasted Bread

On the upside, eggs are not expensive. During the Great Recession of 2008, I befriended eggs, whole grain bread, herbs, and spices for gourmet flavor. So, this wholesome breakfast is a nostalgic treat I enjoyed on days when it was dicey. I added herbal tea and a bit of local honey for all seasons. The sandwich reminded me of mid-week before my parents got paid. We'd often have breakfast for dinner to get through the crunch time. It's also a feel-good, energizing meal, whether you're in the money. Or not. You never know when Lady Luck will cut you a break. (Remember to put a bit of bay leaf in a safe place for bringing you good fortune.)

2 brown eggs (at room temperature)
½ cup 2 percent organic low-fat milk
1 Roma tomato, chopped
    Lemon black pepper to taste
Dash of nutmeg
2 tablespoons cheddar cheese, shredded
½ cup tomatoes, cherry, sliced
Parsley, basil, or thyme sprigs, fresh (for garnish)
2 slices whole grain bread, toasted

Whisk eggs and milk. Pour into a nonstick frying pan. Cook on medium heat. Stir as needed till eggs are cooked and fluffy. Add chopped tomato. Sprinkle with pepper and dash of nutmeg. Grate fresh cheese on top. Garnish with tomatoes and herbs. Serve on top of whole grain toast.

Serves 1 or 2.

Tossed Salad With Creamy Garlic Dressing

In the mid-1970s, salads were my chosen grub for lunch and dinner. The macrobiotic trend was "in" along with running, yoga, hot tubs, and saunas. It was the sign of the times to healthy up to get and stay lean. This basic salad is a no brainer—but the herbed dressing, gifted by Eden Foods, is a special garlicky delight that I enjoy.

6 cups mixed baby salad greens
1 medium cucumber, sliced into rounds
3 medium organic tomatoes, sliced into wedges
1 cup red onion, sliced into thin half-rings

DRESSING

¼ cup Eden Extra Virgin Olive Oil
¼ cup water
1 tablespoon Eden Yellow Mustard
⅛ teaspoon Eden Sea Salt, or to taste
2 cloves garlic, minced or pressed
¼ cup scallions, thinly sliced
2 tablespoons fresh parsley, minced or pressed
2 teaspoons organic maple syrup, optional
1 tablespoon Eden Red Wine Vinegar

Place all dressing ingredients in a blender and blend until creamy. Arrange salad vegetables on individual plates and spoon dressing over.

Serves 6.

(Courtesy: Eden Foods)

Vegetable Shell Pasta Salad With Olives, Fennel, & Onions

Pasta salad has countless variations, from the type of pasta used and choice of herbs. This recipe is provided by Eden Foods. I chose to include it because they put fennel to work and roast garlic, which is fascinating. The effort put into this pasta salad is worth the time because the flavors are amazing.

12 ounces Eden Vegetable Shells
1 fennel bulb, cut in half, then sliced into half moons
1 large onion, sliced into half moons
2 cloves garlic, do not peel
2 teaspoons Eden Extra Virgin Olive Oil
1½ cups organic tomatoes, diced
¾ cup pitted Kalamata olives, sliced, or sliced pitted
*   black olives*
½ cup fresh basil, chopped, or fresh chopped parsley,
*   or dill*

DRESSING

⅓ cup Eden Extra Virgin Olive Oil
⅓ cup Eden Red Wine Vinegar
2 tablespoon lemon juice, freshly squeezed
½ teaspoon Eden Sea Salt
⅛ teaspoon freshly ground black pepper

Preheat the oven to 425 degrees F. Cook pasta per package directions, drain, rinse, and set aside. Toss fennel, onion, and whole garlic with 2 teaspoons olive oil. Spread on baking sheet and roast in oven until tender, 20 to 30 minutes. Remove and set aside. In a bowl, whisk together oil, vinegar, lemon juice, salt, and pepper. Squeeze roasted garlic out of its peel, dice, and whisk into dressing. In a bowl toss roasted vegetable with pasta. Add tomatoes, olives, herbs, and dressing. Toss, and serve as is or cover and refrigerate and serve as cold salad.

Serves 8.

(Courtesy: Eden Foods)

ENTREES

Chicken with Saffron Rice
Garlicky Turkey Stuffed Bell Peppers
Herby Tostadas with Cilantro Sauce
Roasted Paprika Cornish Hens
Spicy Italian Meatballs

The main dish of a meal is often the served food that gets the most recognition for dinner. The fascinating thing is the types of herbs and spices used can change up a dish, giving it flavors and a distinct type of cuisine. Different herbs and spices can make a fish presentation Asian, Indian, Mediterranean, Mexican, or whatever type of cuisine fits your fancy. Yes, using the right amount of seasoning can make a dish—and the chefs and judges on the Food Network channel often tell the audience just that. Let's say you have fresh salmon. Add parsley and thyme and it's an Italian plate. Go for Cajun spices and you're south of the border. Mix it up with turmeric and you've got a little bit of India. See how important herbs and spices and your choices can be in cooking?

Chicken with Saffron Rice

The Spice House will tell you a small dose of heaven and an emblem of the historic Silk Road is in Rumi's premier saffron. Saffron, sourced from Afghan farmers, is the inspiration of this simple but unforgettable side dish. It's more exotic than plain white rice you are served in a take-out box of Chinese cuisine or brown rice boiled at home to pair with crucifers. It's time to go out of the comfort zone and enjoy another spice of life.

3 cups water
1 small onion, diced
5–6 tablespoons cooking oil (preferably olive oil)
Salt to taste
¼ teaspoon ground cardamom
1 teaspoon cumin
½ cup golden raisins
2 cups basmati rice
Toasted almond, pistachio, or pine nuts, for garnish

In a large pot or teakettle, bring 3 cups of water to a slow boil. In another large pot, fry onions in oil on medium high heat, adding salt, cardamom, and cumin. Stir until the spices coat the onions. Cook until glassy, but not quite caramelized, stirring as needed. Remove the onions when they are ready, reduce heat, then fry raisins in the same manner, adding more oil if needed. Be careful not to burn the raisins, as they have a high sugar content. When the raisins have puffed up, remove them and set aside with the onions.

Rinse rice in room temperature water, so as to remove any excess starch. Let as much water drain off the rice before lightly frying in about 2 tablespoons oil. This will give the rice a toasted and nutty flavor. In a small cup, put your saffron in ½ cup water and set aside. Add the other 2¼ cups of hot water to the rice, use a spoon to make sure no rice is sticking to the pot. Salt your water to taste.

Once the rice and water are simmering, add onions, raisins, and saffron water. Make sure to get all the threads into the rice. Stir until onions, raisins, and saffron are fully incorporated. Cover with lid just slightly off kilter so steam can slowly waft away. Slowly steam the rice for 5 to 10 minutes or until desired texture is reached. Be careful not to over stir the rice as basmati is fragile when cooked and will break apart. Serve in your favorite bowl, and garnish with a few threads of dried saffron. Garnish with toasted almond, pistachio, or pine nuts.

Helpful hints: For a more subtle flavor, you can substitute the cumin and cardamom for coriander. Use yellow or white onion, as red onions will distract from the saffron's vibrant color. You can use black cardamom or the more popular green cardamom.

Serves 4 to 5.

(Courtesy: The Spice House)

Garlicky Turkey Stuffed Bell Peppers

One Thanksgiving holiday I took an alternative route instead of cooking a big turkey. I turned to ground turkey, bell peppers, and plenty of herbs and spices. Nah, it wasn't a traditional dinner but it was festive and flavorful. Also, Stuffed Bell Peppers were a popular recipe when I was growing up. Nowadays, as an adult who liked the peppers, I tweak it with a twenty-first-plant, based-century touch.

4 bell peppers, green or red
¼ cup olive oil
2 garlic cloves, chopped

1 onion, yellow, chopped
8 ounces turkey, lean, ground
½ cup seasoned breadcrumbs
½ cup Romano cheese, grated
¼ up Monterey Jack cheese, shredded
1 egg, organic, brown
¼ cup pine nuts
½ cup parsley, fresh, chopped
2 teaspoons Mediterranean Seasoning (Mountain Rose
    Herbs)
Sliced tomatoes and Parm cheese, grated for garnish

Preheat the oven to 350 degrees F. Slice tops of peppers, remove seeds. Save or toss tops. Set aside. In a large frying pan, on medium heat, add oil, garlic, onion, and turkey. Stir until cooked. Remove from stovetop. Set aside. In a bowl add breadcrumbs, cheese, egg, nuts, parsley, and spice blend. Stuff the mixture into peppers. Place pepper tops on peppers or not. Put in an 8-inch by 8-inch baking dish filled with about 1 cup water. Place a piece of foil on top. Bake for about 50 minutes. Remove from oven. Top with tomato slices and cheese.

Serves 4.

Herby Tostadas with Cilantro Sauce

Meatless tostadas are an easy dish to make and one of my favorites. Cilantro sauce gives these gems a spicy flavor and healthful kick. It's an ideal recipe to use in the spring or summer because it's quick and satisfying without spending too much time in the kitchen. Perfect for an outdoor meal.

2 flour tortillas, whole wheat honey oat
1 teaspoon extra virgin olive oil
1 cup kale mix, pre-shredded and packaged
2 tablespoons red onion, chopped
Olive oil and red wine vinegar to taste (3 to 1 ratio of
     oil to vinegar works well)
1 Roma tomato, chopped
½ cup cruciferous vegetables (broccoli, cauliflower)
½ cup cheese, feta, cubed
½ cup salsa with cayenne and garlic, fresh (store-
     bought or from a restaurant)
1 lemon
Parmesan shavings (garnish)
Sour cream (garnish)

CILANTRO SAUCE

¼ cup cilantro
¼ cup basil
1 tablespoon cayenne pepper
¼ cup extra virgin olive oil

In a blender, combine cilantro, basil, cayenne pepper, and oil. Pulse until smooth. Set aside. Place tortillas on a plate. Drizzle with oil. Heat for 1 minute in the microwave. Remove and turn tortilla over. Repeat. It should be crispy. You can oven bake or fry but this is easy and works. Set aside. In a bowl combine kale mix, onion, olive oil and vinegar, and tomato. Set aside. Nuke crucifers in the microwave for a few minutes (or stir-fry with a bit of olive oil in a skillet). Place tostadas on a plate. Top with salad mixture. Top with cheese, salsa, and squeeze a bit of lemon juice on each tostada. Top with shavings and a dollop of sour cream. Drizzle with cilantro sauce.

Serves 2.

Roasted Paprika Cornish Hens

Cornish hens are a fine dish for holidays but can be enjoyed for all seasons. Seasoning the dish up with paprika, rosemary, and thyme leaves made the main dish aromatic and extraordinary. This recipe is inspired by my childhood and it is a gift from an established spice company who gets the art of bringing together flavor, home, and family.

2 whole Cornish hens, about 1¼ pounds each
2 tablespoons olive oil
2 teaspoons McCormick Organic Paprika
2 teaspoons McCormick Organic Rosemary
1 teaspoon McCormick Organic Garlic Powder
1 teaspoon McCormick Gourmet Sicilian Sea Salt
1 teaspoon McCormick Gourmet Organic Thyme
½ teaspoon McCormick Gourmet Organic Black
    Pepper, coarse ground

Preheat the oven to 350 degrees F. Place hens on rack in shallow roasting pan. Brush with oil. Mix paprika, rosemary, garlic powder, sea salt, thyme, and pepper in small bowl. Rub evenly over entire surface of hens. Roast 1 to 1¼ hours until hens are cooked through.

Serves 4.

(Courtesy: McCormick)

Spicy Italian Meatballs

In the eighties, I did cook up meat dishes for my friends, the carnivores. During the twenty-first century, for a Thanksgiving dinner I made the decision to toss the tradition of making a turkey and dressing. Instead, I changed it up and cooked up a main Mediterranean meal complete with spicy turkey meatballs and linguine. It was easy to put together and the herbs and spices, including fennel, cloves, garlic, onions, and nutmeg, made it a memorable feast. Hemingway would be proud, and my guests were wowed.

2 or 3 slices Italian bread
½ pound pork or lamb, lean, ground
½ pound veal or turkey (no skin) ground
½ pound beef, lean, ground
½ cup fresh basil and/or parsley, chopped
½ cup Romano cheese, grated
¾ cup provolone, shredded
Salt, pepper, and cayenne to taste
1 egg and 1 egg white
2 teaspoons anise or fennel seeds
½ cup raisins or currants
¼ cup pine nuts
4 garlic cloves minced
Pinch of cloves, cinnamon, or nutmeg
4 green onions (white part) chopped
⅓ cup Marsala Olive Fruit Oil

Soak bread in water, squeeze water out and crumble into a mixing bowl. And remaining ingredients except oil. Mix very lightly until well blended. Form into meatballs in size desired. Pressing the mixture too tightly will make the meatballs too firm. In large skillet heat olive oil, add meatballs. Cook until brown on all sides.

May have to be cooked in 2 batches over medium heat. Add to gravy, soup, stews, meat pies, and so forth.

Makes 12 to 16.

(Courtesy: Gemma Sanita Sciabica, *Cooking with California Olive Oil: Treasured Family Recipes*)

DESSERTS

Sweet and savory desserts with herbs are one of life's simple pleasures. Well, actually, if both herbs and spices are included, they can be complex with layers of depth. A teacake with its fall spices, such as cinnamon and nutmeg, is a gift. A slice of spiced carrot cake can be sublime as long as cloves and vanilla bean frosting with sprigs of fresh herbs are part of the mix. A creamy custard with saffron notes is an extraordinary treat. Crisps and crumbles with allspice and cardamom can titillate your taste buds in autumn, winter, spring, and summer with the perfect seasonal fruit—and fresh herbs of the season. Desserts like comforting Autumn Allspice Teacake and Nutmeg Peach Crumble for hot summer days can be even more delicious and healthful when garnished with an array of fresh herbs, including basil, lavender, mint, and rosemary.

Autumn Allspice Teacake
Nutmeg Peach Crumble
Orange-Thyme California Cookies
Spice Cake with Prune Filling
Vanilla Cardamom Whoopie Pies
Zesty Carrot Cake with Vanilla Bean Frosting

Autumn Allspice Teacake

My culinary skills during my youth were not much better than a kid playing chef with a toy oven and miniature cake mixes (yes, I did that). Thankfully my skills have improved since I was a teen. It was often a hit-or-miss when I baked because of not following directions. But this apple cake is stress-free and undemanding. Perhaps I can give credit to the simplicity of the recipe—and using the right combination of spices makes it sweet and savory.

1½ cups cake flour
1 cup all-purpose flour
½ cup granulated white sugar
1 cup light brown sugar
2 tablespoons baking soda
1 teaspoon allspice (McCormick)
1 teaspoon cardamom (The Spice House)
2 teaspoons cinnamon-sugar
1 stick European-style butter, soft (save 1 tablespoon
    for greasing pan)
¼ cup half-and-half
2 large eggs
½ cup each apples and plums, fresh, washed, peeled,
    cored, sliced (extra if you want to arrange on top
    for an elegant presentation)
¾ cup caramel chips
¼ cup hazelnuts, chopped (optional)
Confectioners sugar (for dusting)
Caramel sauce, premium brand (for drizzling on top or
    bottom of cake)

Preheat the oven to 325 degrees F. In a bowl, combine flours, sugars, baking soda, and spices. Add the butter, half-and-half, and eggs. Mix well. Fold in apples, plums, caramel chips, and nuts. Spread batter in a 9-inch by 2-inch or a bit larger round baking pan or tart baking dish. Top with apple wedges in a circle design. Bake for approximately 45 minutes or until firm to touch. Remove from oven and cool. Leave in tart dish. Dust with sugar. Cut in slices. Place on plates and drizzle with caramel sauce. Pair it with chamomile tea.

Serves 8 to 10.

Nutmeg Peach Crumble

❖ ❖ ❖

I have had a real like for crumbles since I was a kid. Of all of the seasonal recipes I've used, this one is the one I love most. Give credit to the mix of spices and vibrant green fresh mint for color, aroma, and presentation. Fresh peaches are plentiful in California to the Deep South in the summertime—and the juicy fruit makes this recipe come alive, especially with all the spices.

2 cups peaches, fresh and sliced
½ cup white granulated sugar
¼ cup all-purpose flour
1 teaspoon cinnamon
¼ teaspoon cardamom
1 teaspoon allspice

TOPPING

¾ cup self-rising flour
¼ cup European-style butter, melted
½ cup brown sugar
1 teaspoon cinnamon-sugar
¼ cup oats
¼ teaspoon nutmeg
Whipped cream or vanilla gelato
Sprigs of fresh mint or thyme

Preheat the oven to 350 degrees F. In a bowl, combine peaches, sugar, flour, and spices. Put mixture into ramekins. Place in baking dish filled halfway with water. Top with mixture of flour, butter, sugars, oats, and nutmeg. Bake about 30 to 40 minutes until the topping is golden brown and peaches are bubbly and tender. Serve warm. Top with a dollop of whipped cream or vanilla gelato. Garnish with fresh mint or thyme.

Serves 4.

Orange-Thyme California Cookies

The first morning awakening in Alaska I discovered fresh oranges and juice is non-existent in December. These treasures are MIA to Alaskans in the wintertime. (Note: Reindeer sausages are on their menus.) Once back home in Northern California, I stocked my kitchen counters and fridge with fresh oranges, grapefruits, and lemons from throughout the Golden State. Then, I made a batch of fresh orange-thyme cookies.

1 stick European-style butter, softened
¼ cup confectioners sugar (about ½ cup extra for
*   rolling after baked)*
1 cup all-purpose flour, sifted
2 capfuls pure vanilla extract
¼ cup fresh squeezed orange juice
1 teaspoon orange rind, grated
1 teaspoon fresh or dried thyme, crushed leaves
¼–½ cup nuts (walnuts), chopped

Preheat the oven to 350 degrees F. In a bowl, cream butter and sugar. Add flour and mix until creamy. Stir in vanilla and orange juice. Fold in rind, thyme, and nuts.

Place cookie dough on a floured cutting board and roll into a ball. Put onto a sheet of foil and into the refrigerator for about 20 minutes. Take out, place on a cutting board. Use a small ice cream scoop (about -cup size) and scoop dough into balls. Roll into a ball shape and place on nonstick cookie sheet or lined with parchment paper. Bake for 12 minutes or until bottom of cookies are light brown. Do not overbake. Place balls into sugar immediately. After cooled repeat. Serve with herbal tea or coffee with infused spices.

Makes 8–10. You can double the recipe as well as freeze the cookies in an airtight container.

Spice Cake with Prune Filling

In the twentieth century, easy-to-use store-bought cake mixes were a huge trend. But TV chefs and major cookbook authors dished up homemade recipes for baking cakes, like this one. I recall in my junior high Home Economics class we had a baking contest. It was the homemade mocha log that won; my Boston Cream Pie got a mention. If I could go back in time, I would recreate this spice cake to win the judging teacher's palate. This recipe was created by my talented longtime central California friend, co-owner of Sciabica's Olive Oil.

3 egg whites
1½ cups sugar, divided
2 cups flour
3 tablespoons baking powder
½ teaspoon salt
1 teaspoon nutmeg
¼ teaspoon cloves
¼ teaspoon cardamom
1½ teaspoons cinnamon

1 tablespoon molasses
¼ cup Marsala Olive Fruit Oil
⅔ cup milk
3 egg yolks
2 teaspoons vanilla

Preheat the oven to 350 degrees F. Grease and flour two 9-inch by 1½-inch cake pans. Beat egg whites in a bowl until foamy. Add slowly ½ cup sugar. Beat until whites hold stiff peaks. In a mixing bowl add flour, remaining 1 cup sugar, baking powder, salt, and spices. Make a well in the center and add molasses, olive oil, milk, yolks, and vanilla. Blend. Fold in very gently beaten egg whites. Pour into prepared pans, bake for 25 to 30 minutes. Remove from pans, cool on rack. Slice each cake into 2 layers. Set aside.

SPICED PRUNE FILLING

The splendor of this cake is that prunes are elegant but you can substitute the fruit with dates and walnuts or pecans. Whatever fruit or nut you use, the spices will provide decadent flavor and make this spice cake one to use for a special occasion. If you choose, leave the top plain but dust it with confectioners sugar—the spice filling will be a surprise touch.

3 cups heavy cream
½ cup confectioners sugar (or to taste)
1 tablespoon ginger liqueur
1½ teaspoons cinnamon
¾ teaspoon nutmeg
¼ teaspoon cloves
1½ cups finely chopped, cooked, pitted prunes
2 ounces milk chocolate, room temperature

In large mixing bowl, whip cream. Add sugar, liqueur, and spices. To whipped cream mixture, very gently fold in well drained, chopped prunes. Spread ¼ cup prune filling on each layer ending with top. Sides need not be frosted. To make chocolate curls use a vegetable peeler. Decorate with chocolate curls sprinkled around outer edges of top layer. Keep refrigerated until ready to serve.

Serves 12.

(Courtesy: Gemma Sanita Sciabica, *Baking with California Olive Oil: Dolci and Biscotti Recipes*)

Vanilla Cardamom Whoopie Pies

A classic favorite—a "Whoopie Pie," which was founded in the 1920s, becomes an comfort food dessert when infused with aromatic cardamom and familiar vanilla flavor. Take a look at this decadent treat where East meets West from yesteryear to present-day.

COOKIES

2 cups flour
½ cup unsweetened cocoa powder
1¼ teaspoons baking soda
1 teaspoon salt
¼ teaspoon McCormick Gourmet Organic Cardamom, ground
1 cup buttermilk
1 teaspoon McCormick Gourmet Organic Premium Pure Vanilla Extract
½ cup (1 stick) butter, softened
1 cup firmly packed brown sugar
1 egg

Vanilla Cardamom Filling

½ cup (1 stick) butter, softened
1½ cups confectioners sugar
1½ cups marshmallow cream
2 teaspoons McCormick Gourmet Organic Premium
 Pure Vanilla Extract
¼ teaspoon McCormick Organic Cardamom, ground
⅓ cup finely chopped salted shelled pistachios

For the cookies, preheat the oven to 350 degrees F. Mix flour, cocoa powder, baking soda, salt, and cardamom in medium bowl; set aside. Mix buttermilk and vanilla in medium bowl. Set aside. Mix buttermilk and vanilla in small bowl. Beat butter and brown sugar in large bowl with electric mixer on medium-high speed until light and fluffy. Add egg; mix well. Add flour mixture alternately with buttermilk mixture, beating on low speed after each addition until smooth and scraping down sides of bowl occasionally. Spoon 1 tablespoon of batter, 2 inches apart, onto parchment paper-lined large baking sheets. (Cookies will spread so avoid crowding them on baking sheet.) Bake 8 minutes or until cookies are puffed and spring back when touched, turning baking sheets halfway through baking. Cool on baking sheets 1 minute. Remove to wire racks; cool completely.

For the filling, beat butter, confectioners sugar, marshmallow cream, vanilla, and cardamom in medium bowl with electric mixer on medium speed until light and fluffy. To assemble the Whoopie Pies, place 1 tablespoon filling on flat side of 1 cookie. Top with a second cookie, pressing gently to spread the filling. Repeat with remaining cookies. Roll edge of cookies in chopped pistachios. Store whoopie pies between layers of wax paper in airtight container in refrigerator up to 5 days.

Makes approximately 6 to 12 depending on the size you prefer.

(Courtesy: McCormick)

Zesty Carrot Cake with Vanilla Bean Frosting

❖ ❖ ❖

Carrot cake goes back centuries. Food historians believe it has roots of carrot pudding consumed by Europeans in the Middle Ages. In the twentieth century it made its way to North America. Filled with warming spices, such as allspice, cinnamon, cloves, nutmeg, and topped with a vanilla bean frosting makes it a seasoned masterpiece for autumn or winter. Also, for a lighter springtime or Easter cake, forgo the frosting and garnish with fresh herb sprigs.

1¾ cups flour (cake flour)
⅔ cup all-purpose flour
2 teaspoons baking soda
1½ teaspoons cinnamon
¾ teaspoon ginger or nutmeg
¼ teaspoon ground cloves or allspice
½ teaspoon salt
1 cup brown sugar, packed
½ cup European-style butter, unsalted
2 eggs
⅔ cup buttermilk
1 teaspoon pure vanilla extract
3 cups organic carrots, shredded
½ cup raisins, golden
⅓ cup walnuts, finely chopped

Preheat the oven to 350 degrees F. Grease a 13-inch by 9-inch by 2-inch baking pan. In mixing bowl add dry ingredients, flours, baking soda, spices, and sugar. Make well in center. Stir in butter, eggs, buttermilk, and vanilla. Fold in carrots, raisins, and nuts. Pour batter into prepared pan. Bake 35 to 40 minutes or until cake tester comes out clean from center. Cool completely in pan on wire rack.

Makes 12 squares.

Vanilla Bean Cream Cheese Frosting

❖ ❖ ❖

1 cup cream cheese, softened
2 tablespoons European-style butter
¼ cup whole milk
1 teaspoon pure vanilla extract (or use vanilla bean
*   paste)*
1 teaspoon fennel, ground (The Spice House)
Walnuts, chopped for garnish
Sprigs of fresh lavender, mint, rosemary, or thyme

In a bowl, combine cream cheese, 2 tablespoons butter, ¼ cup whole milk, 1 teaspoon pure vanilla extract. Blend until creamy. Fold in fennel. Frost top of cake. Garnish with walnuts and sprigs of herbs of your choice.

HEALING HIGHLIGHTS FROM NATURE'S GARDEN-FEST

✓ Savoring different herbs and spices in foods at restaurants, cafés, food stands, and trucks gives you a taste of adventure—eating on the wild seasoned side.
✓ Experimenting with fresh and dried herbs in homemade dishes can be fun, exciting, and add a little more zest and healing powers to foods.
✓ Using premium herbs and spices is the way to go so you can enjoy the best herbs and spices experience.
✓ Be bold! Be fearless! Be spontaneous! Try new-ish herbs and spices, including store-bought and DIY blends. Yes, discover ancient herbs and spices are the variety of life.

FINAL WORDS OF HERBAL WISDOM

Herbs and spices play a big role in life and well-being. When my solo expedition to Alaska aka "The Last Frontier" finally happened, I anticipated fresh and exciting seasonings, northern lights, and a moose sighting. Sometimes, fantasies are healthier than real life . . .

In Anchorage at 9:00 A.M., I sat in my hotel room bed on the seventeenth floor overlooking downtown, and Chugach Mountains— but it was dark. I called room service. No freshly squeezed orange juice with fresh mint sprigs or coffee lattes with fresh spices. You will not likely find garden-fresh herbal treasures in December. Blame it on the lack of sunlight. Fresh food is expensive if it's imported. And that's not all . . .

HERBAL DELIGHTS

The last night I was nursing a sore throat. I ordered a Greek pizza. It had chunks of real garlic! Another herbal highlight of the Alaska adventure was finding an artisan chocolate shop. I bought a peri-cayenne pepper truffle, caramelized pear saffron chocolate, and a white square of chocolate with pink peppercorn. The cayenne and dark chocolate gave me the gift of those feel-good endorphins and soothed my raw throat that hurt when swallowing. Both garlic and cayenne made me feel better.

MY SEASONED CABIN

On the upside: I'm no longer thinking the herbal grass is greener in Alaska, a place where fresh food is not abundant year-round. But dried herbs, such as the parsley, pepper, and paprika on French fries, did suffice. Drinking plenty of herbal tea made me less homesick and more welcome. Sometimes, you have to go out of your comfort zone to gain hands-on knowledge.

While Dr. Will Clower was sailing around the world enjoying different cuisines, cultures, and fresh seasonings on board his vessel and off at exotic ports—I was in the air and on land enduring erratic weather and foraging dried herbs and spices in a hotel.

The thing that kept us connected is that we both followed our passion. We are both modern-day pioneers and followers of the Mediterranean diet and lifestyle. And one of the benefits is experiencing timeless treasures—valuable seasonings—which you, too, encounter whether at home or have been bit by the nomadic spirit.

So, you have my kitchen table wisdom of herbs and spices. The best part: When you want to use an herbal recipe to eat, for beauty, or our home, I am your tour guide 24/7. It took a trip to Alaska for me to appreciate the timeless treasures that I have right at home inside my cabin.

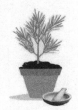

PART 7

HERBS AND SPICES
RESOURCES

Herbs and Spices Resources: Where Can You Buy Seasonings?

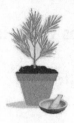

HERBS AND SPICES BRANDS

Mountain Rose Herbs
P.O. Box 50220
Eugene, OR 97405
www.mountainroseherbs.com

Founded in 1987, an array of herbs and spices.

Plant Therapy
510 2nd Avenue S
Twin Falls, ID 83301
www.plantherapy.com

A wide array of essential oils, roll-on blends, carrier oils, KidSafe products, aromatic jewelry, and more.

The Great American Spice Co.
10451 Northland Drive NE
Rockford, MI 49341
www.americanspice.com

The Spice House
1512 N. Wells Street
Chicago, IL
thespicehouse.com

Specialty Foods with Herbs and Spices

Lake Champlain Chocolates
750 Pine Street
Burlington, VT 05401
www.lakechamplainchocolates.com

Dark Spicy Aztec Chocolate Bar. Blended from semisweet dark chocolate, crunchy pumpkin seeds, hot cayenne pepper, and cinnamon.

Nick Sciabica & Sons
2150 Yosemite Boulevard
Modesto, CA 95354
www.sunshineinabottle.com

Sciabica specializes in cold-pressed olive oils using varieties of California olives.

National Health Organizations

American Cancer Society
www.cancer.org

American Heart Association
www.heart.org

NATIONAL FOOD ORGANIZATIONS

North American Olive Oil Association
3301 Route 66, Suite 205, Building C
Neptune, NJ 07753
www.naooa.org

This association is committed to supplying North America consumers with quality products in a fair and competitive environment; providing some recipes with herbs, spices, and olive oil.

HERB ORGANIZATIONS

The Herb Society of America
9019 Kirkland-Chardon Road
Kirkland, OH 44094
www.herbsociety.org

An organization that includes plenty of in-depth information on herbs including cultivation, herb and pollinator conservation, and even topics "beyond the garden," such as herbal wellness, their library features herbs, and DIY projects.

HERBAL COFFEE AND TEA RETAILERS

Here are a few of my favorite tea brands and a new one that I discovered during my journey in the land of herbs and spices. Keep in mind, while I recommend these fine companies, there are other brands at your grocery store and online.

Door County Coffee & Tea Co.
www.doorcountycoffee.com

An array of flavored coffees, including Autumn Spice with artificial and natural flavorings of nutmeg and cloves.

Harney & Sons Fine Teas
5723 Route 22
Millerton, NY 12546
www.harney.com

An amazing assortment of herbal and spice teas and tisanes, impressive presentation of each item. A black tea with orange and cloves is fabulous for autumn and winter.

HEALTH SPAS

Cal-a-Vie Health Spa
29402 Spa Havens Way
Vista, CA 92084
www.cal-a-vie.com

Herbs and spices are nothing new as you know. The thing is, they are making a big comeback for many reasons. Remember, spicing it up in meals can help us want to eat less unhealthy trans fats, salt, and sugar—three culprits in the twenty-first-century diet. Also, multigenerations are seeking adventurous grub in this day and age. Flavorful dishes using clean, plant-based foods is what is bringing plant power to the forefront.

Understanding why and how to use herbs and spices is helpful for your mind and body. Companies offer fresh organic herbs and spices but don't ignore dried goods either—both are healthful.

There are dozens of companies, big and small, that offer a wide assortment of herbs and spices. It's your choice. However, do your homework. Find out if their products are organic, where they are sourced, and if they include preservatives or chemicals.

The companies I interviewed are well established. But sometimes, companies merge or change things up. So, if you cannot find a specific brand of one herb or spice—chill. Simply move on to another company and I assure you that you'll get what you need. I gave you a working herb and spice rack collection to expand your knowledge. The rest is up to you. Yes, you can grow your garden-fest outdoors and indoors. Herbs and spices have a long shelf life. But remember to replenish your timeless treasures so they are fresh and flavorful.

Down-to-Earth Glossary

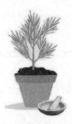

Adaptogens: Herbs that can bolster the immune system. Adaptogens include garlic and thyme.

Analgesics: Herbs that can lessen pain. They include cilantro and cloves.

Antibacterial: Blocks germs from producing. They include garlic and turmeric.

Antidepressant: Reduces sadness, hopelessness. They include marjoram and oregano.

Antifungal: Guards against fungus.

Anti-inflammatory: Lessens irritation, redness, soreness in a variety of body ailments.

Antiseptic: Germ fighting.

Ayurveda: Ancient Indian medicine of the health of mind and body.

Capsaicin: A property found in cayenne that gives them heat and healing powers.

Carcinogenic: Having potential to cause cancer.

Chlorophyll: An ingredient that gives herbs a green color.

Copper: A trace mineral, aids in making collagen for bone and connective tissue.

Exfoliant: Any ingredient whose purpose is to zap dead cells from the skin's surface. Herbal store-bought exfoliants are available or you can create your own.

Flavonoids: Disease fighters that may help to stave off allergies, inflammation; antioxidants may lessen the risk of developing cancer and heart disease.

Herbalism: The study of plant therapy in alternative medicine.

Inflammation: A factor in most health ailments and progressive diseases.

Manganese: A trace mineral to maintain bone formation.

Milliliter. It is abbreviated as mL or ml. A liquid measurement in the metric system. It is used for measuring essential oils, which are extracted from herbs.

Nervines: Herbs that may relax the nervous system. They include allspice and anise.

ORAC value: Oxygen radical absorbance capacity; a ranking for antioxidant amounts.

Phenols: Plant compounds that act as disease-fighting antioxidants.

Polyphenols: Potent antioxidants; include flavonoids, and other plant compounds with disease-fighting properties.

Roller Balls. A glass tube with a roller on top. It's an easy-to-use device to apply essential oils extracted from herbs on the skin.

Stimulants: Herbs and spices believed to boost physiological functions of the body and mind. They include cayenne.

Thymol: An aromatic compound is thyme that is responsible for its health advantages.

Vitamin D: A fat-soluble vitamin guards against bone loss by aiding in the absorption of calcium from the intestinal tract.

Notes

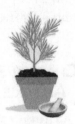

CHAPTER 1:
THE SPICE OF LIFE!

1. Jonny Bowden, Ph.D., 150 Healthiest Foods on Earth, Revised Edition: The Surprising Unbiased Truth about What You Should Eat and Why. Beverly, MA: Fair Winds Press, 2017, page 296.
2. Michael Stroot, The Golden Door Cooks Light & Easy. Layton, UT: Gibbs Smith, 2003, page 29.
3. Ilang T. Alan, "Health Benefits of Culinary Herbs and Spices: Ingent Connect." Journal of AOAC International 102 (2) (March–April 2019): 395–411. DOI: https://doi.org/10.5740/jaoacint.18-0418.
4. Ibid.
5. Common Foods and Flavors of the Mediterranean Diet Pyramid, 2009 Oldways Preservation & Exchange Trust. www.oldwayspt.org.

Chapter 2:
Roots of Plant Power

1. Saul Haley et al., "Phytoliths in Pottery Reveal the Use of Spice in European Prehistoric Cuisine." PLoS ONE (8) (2013): e70583. DOI: 10.1371/journal. pone.0070583.
2. Christine M. Kaefer and John A. Milner, "The Roles of Herbs and Spices in Cancer Prevention." J Nutr Biochem 19 (6) (June 2008): 347–361. DOI:10. 1016/nutbio2007.11.003.

Chapter 3:
Allspice

1. Marjorie Shaffer, Pepper: A History of the World's Most Influential Spice. New York: St. Martin, August 2014, pages 4, 5, 13, 14.
2. Nagarajarao Shamaladevi et al., "Ericifolin: A Novel Antitumor Compound from Allspice That Silences Androgen Receptor in Prostate Cancer." Carcinogenesis34 (8) (August 2013): 1822–1832. Published online 2013 Apr 8. DOI: 10.1093/carcin/bgt123.

Chapter 4:
Anise

1. S. Ashraffodin Ghoshegir et al., "Pimpinella anisum in the Treatment of Functional Dyspepsia: A Double-Blind, Randomized Clinical Trial." J Res Med Sci 20 (1) (January 2015): 13–21.
2. Ibid.

Chapter 5:
Bay Leaf

1. Alam Khan et al., "Bay Leaves Improve Glucose and Lipid Profile of People with Type 2 Diabetes." J Clin Biochem Nutr 44 (1) (January 2009): 52–56. Published online 2008 Dec 27. DOI: 10.3164/jcbn.08-188.

CHAPTER 11:
CLOVES

1. Compound Interest Explorations of everyday chemical compounds, https://www.compoundchem.com/2014/03/13/chemical-compounds-in-herbs-spices/.
2. D. Peixoto-Neves, "Eugenol Dilates Mesenteric Arteries and Reduces Systemic Bp by Activating Endothelial Cell TRPV4 Channels." Br J Pharmacol 172 (14) (July 2015): 3484–3494. DOI: 10.1111/bph.13156.

CHAPTER 13:
DILL

1. "Phytochemical Screening, Antidepressant and Analgesic Effects of Aqueous Extract of Anethum graveolens L., et al." Am J Ther 23 (6) (November/December 2016): e1695–e1699.

CHAPTER 14:
FENNEL

1. Wen-RuiDiao et al., "Chemical Composition, Antibacterial Activity and Mechanism of Action of Essential Oil from Seeds of Fennel (Foeniculum vulgar Mill) Food Control." 35 (2014): 109–116. http://doi.org/10.106/j.foodcont.2013.06.056.
2. Manazoor A. Rather et al., "Foeniculum vulgare: A Comprehensive Review of Its Traditional Use Phytochemistry, Pharmacology, and Safety." Arab J Chem 9 (2) (November 2016): S1574–S1583.
3. M. Ghanzanfarpou et al., "Effect of Foeniculum vulgare (Fennel) on Symptoms of Depression and Anxiety in Postmenopausal Women: A Double-Blind Randomized Controlled Trial." J Obstet Gynaecol 38 (1) (January 2018): 121–126. DOI: 10. 1080/01443615. 2017.1342229.

CHAPTER 15:
GARLIC

1. Gauri Desai et al., "Onion and Garlic Intake and Breast Cancer, a Case-Control Study in Puerto Rico." Nutr Cancer (2019): 1. DOI: 10.1080/01635581.2019.1651349.
2. Patrick Quillin, Ph.D., RD, CNS, Amazing Honey, Garlic, & Vinegar Home Remedies & Recipes. North Canton, OH: The Leader Co., 1996, page 86.

CHAPTER 16:
MARJORAM

1. Hazem S. Elshafie et al., "An Overview of the Biological Effects of Some Mediterranean Essential Oils on Human Health." Biomed Res Int 2017 (2017): 9268468. DOI: 10.1155/2017/9268468.

CHAPTER 17:
NUTMEG

1. Ehad A. Abourashed and Abir T. El-Alfy, "Chemical Diversity and Pharmacological Significance of the Secondary Metabolites of Nutmeg (Myristica fragrans Houtl)." Photochem Rev 14 (6) (December 2016): 1035–1056.
2. Celia Martins et al., "Myristicin from Nutmeg Induces Apoptosis in the Mitochondrial Pathway and Down Regulates Genes of the DNA Damage Response Pathways via the Human Leukemia K562 cells, Chemo-Biological Interactions." Chem Biol Interact 218 (25) (July 2014): 1–9. https://DOI: org/10.1016/j.cbi.2014.04.014.
3. Xiao-NanYang et al., "PPARa Mediates the Hepatoprotective Effects of Nutmeg." Journal of Proteome Research 17 (5) (2018): 1887–1897. DOI: 10.1021.acs.jproteome.7600901.

CHAPTER 18:
OREGANO

1. Jonny Bowden, Ph.D., 150 Healthiest Foods on Earth, Revised Edition: The Surprising Unbiased Truth about What You Should Eat and Why. Beverly, MA: Fair Winds Press, 2007, page 287.

CHAPTER 19:
PAPRIKA

1. Sheila G. West et al., "Spices and Herbs May Improve Cardiovascular Risk Factors." Nutrition Today,49 (5) (September/October 2014): 58–59: S8. DOI: 10.1097/01.NT.0000453846.91592.ca.

CHAPTER 20:
PARSLEY

1. Victor V. Semenov et al., "Efficient Synthesis of Glaziovianin A Isoflavone Series from Dill and Parsley Extracts and Their in Vitro/in Vivo Antimitotic Activity." J Nat Prod (2016). DOI: 10.1021/acs.jnatprod.6b00173.

CHAPTER 21:
SAFFRON

1. Sabna Kotta et al., "Exploring Scientifically Proven Herbal Aphrodisiacs." Pharma Cogn Rev7 (13) (January–June 2013):1–10. www.ncbi.nlm.nih.gov/pmc/articles/PMC3731873/. Last accessed November 19, 2019.

CHAPTER 23:
THYME

1. C. Ely, "Potential Therapeutic Effects of Phytochemical and Medicinal Herbs for Cancer Prevention and Treatment." Arc Gen

Intern Med 2 (3) (2018). www.alliedacademies.org/archives-of-general-internalmedicine/ISSN: 259-7951.

Chapter 24:
Turmeric

1. C. Di Lorenzo, M. Dell'Agli, M. Badea, et al., "Plant Food Supplements with Anti-Inflammatory Properties: A Systematic Review (II)." Crit Rev Food Sci Nutr 53 (5) (2013): 507–516.

Chapter 26:
Season Up, Slim Down

1. R. Zae et al., "Effect of Cumin Powder and Body Composition and Lipid Profile in Overweight and Obese Women." Complement Ther Clin Pract 20 (4) (November 2014): 297–301. DOI: 10.1016/j.ctcp. 2014. 10.001./Epub 2014 Oct 12.
2. Maryam Mashmoul et al., "Saffron: A Natural Potent Antioxidant as a Promising Anti-Obesity Drug." Antioxidants 2 (4) (December 2014): 293–308.

Chapter 27:
Longevity on the Rack

1. M. Frances, K. Williams, et al., "Dietary Garlic and Hip Osteoarthritis: Evidence of a Protective Effect and Putative Mechanism of Action." BMC Musculoskeletal Disord 11 (1) (2010): 280 DOI: 10. 1186/1471-2474-11-280.

Chapter 28:
Herbal Healings from the Garden

1. Jonathan A. Berstein et al., "A Randomized Double-Blind, Parallel Trial Comparing Capsaicin Nasal Spray with Placebo in Subjects with Significant Component of Nonallergic Rhinitis." Ann Allergy

Asthma Immunol 107 (2) (2011): 171–178. DOI: 10:1016/j.an ai. 2011.15.016.

2. C. Cianchetti, "Capsaicin Jelly Against Migraine Pain." Int J Clin Pract 65 (2010): 457–459.

3. Mahshid Bokaie et al., "Oral Fennel (Foeniculum vulgare) Drop Effect On Primary Dysmenorrhea: Effectiveness of Herbal Drug." Iran J Nurs Midwifery Res 18 (2) (March 2013): 128–132.

4. Fatemeh Rahimikian et al., "Effect of Foeniculum vulgar mill (Fennel) on Menopausal Symptoms in Postmenopausal Women." Menopause 24 (9) (September 2017): 1018–1021.

Selected Bibliography

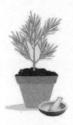

Bowden, Jonny, Ph.D., C.N.S. The 150 Healthiest Foods on Earth: The Surprising Unbiased Truth about What You Should Eat and Why. Beverly, MA: Fair Winds Press, 2017.

Havens, Terri, and John, Chef Curtis Cooke. Beautiful Living: Cooking the Cal-A-Vie Health Spa Way. Vista, CA: Cal-a-Vie, 2019.

Sciabica, Gemma Sanita. Baking with California Olive Oil: Dolci and Biscotti Recipes. Modesto, CA: Gemma Sanita Sciabica, 2002.

Sciabica, Gemma Sanita. Cooking with California Olive Oil: Popular Recipes. Modesto, CA: Gemma Sanita Sciabica, 2001.

Sciabica, Gemma Sanita. Cooking with California Olive Oil: Recipes from the Heart for the Heart. Modesto, CA: Gemma Sanita Sciabica, 2009.

Sciabica, Gemma Sanita. Cooking with California Olive Oil: Treasured Family Recipes. Modesto, CA: Gemma Sanita Sciabica, 1998.

Acknowledgments

I want to thank the open-minded herb savvy nutritionists, medical doctors, and researchers.

As always, Dr. Will Clower, CEO, Mediterranean Wellness, was an ongoing inspiration to me while writing the book. His bold sea adventures kept me motivated and excited as I experienced herbs and spices, on land, past and present, in America and Canada.

The dozens of innovative recipes included in this book are created by herb companies, like Mountain Rose Herbs, Cal-a-Vie's spa's chef, Gemma Sciabica, Eden Foods, the North American Olive Oil Association, and many other wonderful people from America and around the globe.

The Herb Society of America was generous to provide permission to share words and quotes from the "Herb of the Month: Did You Know . . ." pages on their website. The organization's knowledge was helpful; it helped me cross-reference historical facts about herbs and spices.

Not to forget the Kensington Publishing team. For twenty years, I've learned that it takes knowledge and wisdom to go through each process of writing and publishing a book. From the idea of a topic, writing, editing, proofing, artwork, and more—I am forever grateful that we all work well together on a project, like this one.

There is no way I can thank each and every person behind The Healing Powers of Herbs and Spices. Why? Because the people from my past and present are never-ending. But please know, if you discover you are in this book, you have my thanks for coming along the journey.

Blessings and light to all of you who helped me enjoy making the fruition of this book happen. And may herbs and spices—wherever you are—be your timeless treasures for adventurous eating, flavorful food, good health, and well-being.

Connect with U⊙s

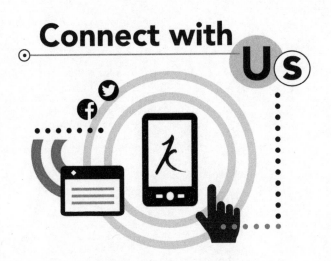

Visit us online at
KensingtonBooks.com
to read more from your favorite authors, see books
by series, view reading group guides, and more.

for sneak peeks, chances to win books and prize packs,
and to share your thoughts with other readers.

facebook.com/kensingtonpublishing
twitter.com/kensingtonbooks

Tell us what you think!

To share your thoughts, submit a review,
or sign up for our eNewsletters, please visit:
KensingtonBooks.com/TellUs.